G000096392

BECOME A RADIANT WOMAN

Hormones In Harmony

BY ROBIN NEEDES

N.D., S.R.N.

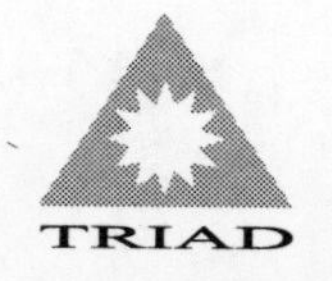

For information address:
TRIAD Publishers Pty.Ltd.
P.O. Box 731
Cairns, Qld. 4870
Australia
Ph: (07) 4093 0121
Fax: (07) 4093 0374
E-mail address: triad@internetnorth.com.au
Web site: http://www.internetnorth.com.au/triad

Book Title:
Become A Radiant Woman
Author:
Robin Needes

National Library Of Australia: ISBN: 0 646 32260 5
Printed in Australia

CONTENTS

To my daughter Victoria Downer
who is a source of loving support
in my life.

Foreword

Every woman should expect to go through her reproductive years without any adverse menstrual symptoms and then flow quite naturally from there into menopause, remaining completely free of problems. This is an inalienable right of all women and one for which we are naturally designed. Unpleasant menstrual and menopausal symptoms mentioned in this book are signs of unbalanced hormones which can be corrected with natural remedies. The hormone imbalance can be so subtle that it does not show up on routine blood tests which only indicate gross imbalances: not the slight changes that can nonetheless create unpleasant mood changes and menstrual irregularities.

A multitude of reasons can be responsible for hormones becoming disordered but most have to do with faulty lifestyles. Stress, poor diets (based on processed, packaged foods), toxic body conditions, nutrient deficiencies and lack of exercise are major causes of hormone imbalance. Emotional problems often have a devastating effect on hormone balance and may be experienced as difficulties in coping with life; a marriage which is not working out, low self-esteem or a lack of time for self to enjoy the healing energy of trees, flowers, meadows, water, sunshine and all types of animal life. Because we are designed by mother nature to self-regulate and self-heal, moment by moment all of our lives, it is important to provide the base materials, a healthy environment and emotional balance for this to occur.

This book is written so every woman may use the tools provided to take control of her own hormone balance by changing her diet and lifestyle and the way in which she reacts to situations which disturb her emotions. In addition, she can utilise the healing properties of plants, vitamins and minerals in order to speed the return to balance. It is such a shame to resort to using brutal methods like surgery to remove the poor suffering organ or to throw hormones at the problem, thus ignoring the body's own innate self-healing mechanism. These are the tools of those who are out of touch with mother nature, of those who do not honour the loving, healing being within womankind. It is surely preferable to experience the joy of taking charge, putting a stop to being a victim of modern medicine and becoming your own healer, secure in the knowledge of your inner power and strength.

To become a radiant woman you must heal your mind, body and spirit by using the gentle tools provided by nature. In this way your hormones will forever remain in harmony and you will be a woman to whom others are instinctively drawn. They will sense your inner grace and beauty and experience peace and harmony in your company. I wish you joy in your journey towards becoming your own medicine woman.

Introduction

This book is written for all women, but especially for those who are in the throes of hormone imbalances or changes. If you are menopausal, pregnant, stressed, suffering from PMT, battling to control your weight or just interested in maintaining good health throughout your life, this is for you. I hope the book will enable you to see the 'big picture' and realise that to cure your problems you need to heal yourself on all levels: physically, emotionally and spiritually.

The book begins with menopause, but there is much for young women to learn in these pages. Indeed, many pages are relevant to all women and to read only the chapter pertaining to your own problem is to miss the book's broad outline. Attempting to deal only with physical cures will mean missing the point that problems may also require emotional healing.

Our eating patterns, thought patterns and emotions all affect our physical bodies and it is crucial to correct imbalances in all of these areas for health to become a reality. Nature has provided us with many tools for physical and emotional healing: homeopathy, herbs, flower essences, essential oils, nutrition and lifestyle changes are the ones I highlight because they are in the realm of my expertise and clinical experience. However, there is a wealth of other healing methods available such as acupuncture, chiropractic or osteopathy, light, colour and crystal healing as well as energy balancing and spiritual healing.

A high percentage of my practice is involved with women's problems that require much more than a prescription Band-Aid. Time is often needed to gently bring the focus to the need for inner searching, feeling negative emotions and shifting them so that a new positive powerful outlook results. The flower essences and homeopathic remedies assist this process, while the vitamins and minerals correct physical impediments to health. Dietary changes are part of the cure and a must for future prevention and good health.

Every woman is unique and no two individuals receive the same treatment. However the tools I use effectively are outlined in this book for the benefit of all women. My own life experiences have enabled me to understand the 'big picture' and I am indebted to the dear friends who guided and supported me in my spiritual awakening and the healing of my life. The severe menopausal symptoms which I experienced initially were a blessing in that they prompted me to examine the many methods of healing for menopausal women and to find the most effective tools within my range of skills. Part of this trail involved discovering that permanent relief comes, not only from using the appropriate remedies on an individual basis, but also from healing the emotional body so that it no longer disturbs the hormone balance.

What I have additionally realised, as an important part of the 'big picture', is that women need to play a major role in the healing of our planet, but to do this we first have to heal our own lives. This patriarchal society in which we have existed for generations has placed women in positions of inferiority, and humanity in an area where weapons are of greater value than living beings. It is nonsense to argue that building and testing vicious means of destruction are necessary to save humanity. This is the deranged thinking of people who are totally out of touch with their higher selves.

It is time for all women to reclaim their inner power and so assist this society which is based on masculine energy towards a balance with feminine intuition. It is time to allow the all-knowing, all-loving feminine energy (intuition) which is part of every man, woman and child, to come forth and become the guiding light for everything we think, say and do. It is time for the intellect (ego) to shift to the position where it implements intuitive knowledge and desire. Herein lies the perfect state for healing ourselves, all humanity and the earth itself.

Our devastated planet, which is a living part of the universal energy field, is so sick it can hardly function. We have choked its rivers with filth in the name of progress, poured unimaginable amounts of refuse into its bowels, blown apart its energy fields with nuclear testing, war and destruction, and taken its energy source by robbing its reserves of coal, crude oil and the gas by-product. This planet of ours is now devastated because we have stolen its means of self-healing. It will cleanse itself by the only method it has left unless we all send healing energy with our actions and thoughts. Negativity must be replaced by love on a world-wide scale - this is how we will turn the tide. Women as the nurturers can lead the way.

Already the earth is endeavouring to cleanse itself - the tidal waves are like a bath to wash away the negativity and the earthquakes are like an attempt to fold all the pollution underneath out of harm's way so that the planet can breathe again. Many thousands of wonderful people are presently involved in either trying to prevent the excesses of our society or actively helping the earth to heal without great upheaval, using the universal energy which all of us can access at any time.

There is great urgency for all of humanity to take part in this exercise so that we can give energy to our beautiful planet to use for its detoxification. Only then will it have the tools of gentle transformation rather than having to use earthquakes and floods to cleanse itself.

So, dear women, let us unite and change our planet into a place of love, respect and compassion for all living things and let us teach others the same values by our example. However, firstly we have to heal our own lives. It is this healing process which enables us to tap into our own inner power and grace and then use these to give love and to light the fuses that will heal humanity and the planet. Dear friend, *you* have this power and there is great urgency for you to use it for the love of all living things.

PART 1 - MENOPAUSE

1. Introducing Menopause

Menopause is a normal phase in a woman's life - even the signs such as hot flushes are normal and not a signal to rush out and get a prescription for hormone replacement therapy, hormones which the body no longer requires. Many women sail through their hormonal changes without any problems and others have slight effects for a short period of time only. Approximately ten percent experience severe symptoms.

Lifestyles, emotions and diets have everything to do with whether the natural flow into menopause is easy or difficult and therefore changes in these areas are the key to reversing any discomfort. Our emotions and diet have major effects on the endocrine glands: the ovaries, adrenals, parathyroids, thyroid and pituitary. Very sensitive women, and particularly those who were shy and blushed easily as a child or teenager, seem to be most prone to menopausal flushes.

With the curtailment of ovulation there is a rise in two hormones from the pituitary gland called the follicle stimulating hormone (FSH) and luteinizing hormone (LH) as they are trying to stimulate the ovaries to release more ova. Once the pituitary gets the message that the ovaries are in permanent retirement FSH and LH levels drop. These two hormones are involved in the hot flushes and night sweats. Those who take hormone replacement therapy (HRT) will often go through menopausal symptoms whenever they try to come off the hormones because the pituitary gland is triggered to over react every time for a period. Once the ovaries retire, the female hormones are produced by the adrenal glands in increasing amounts. If a menopausal woman displays no adverse symptoms, it means that her adrenal glands are secreting female hormones as nature decreed and the follicle stimulating hormone has subsided into retirement.

Our adrenal glands make hormones which control our reactions to stressful situations and as long as we react correctly, the outpouring of hormones ceases when the stress passes. However, many people remain in a state of stress for years on end which in time weakens the adrenal glands to the extent that they cannot function properly. This means that in menopause they may not secrete enough female hormones. If you recognise yourself here, the solution is to deal with the stress (see Part 1, chapter 19) so that your hormone levels return to normal. Taking HRT also causes the adrenal glands to constantly secrete stress hormones which upsets mineral balances and causes a lack of female hormones from this alternative source.

A considerable amount of clinical research into female hormones has been published by Dr. Raymond Peat Ph.D. of the United States and he believes that oestrogen replacement is needed only for a tiny fraction of the population who perhaps suffer serious vaginal dryness. Respected pioneers in hormonal research like Loes and Selye have published a wealth of evidence showing that added oestrogen is actually toxic to the human body. One example is that oestrogen prevents urinary loss of excessive blood calcium. Instead this calcium is deposited as crystals in joints and soft tissue and this is clearly harmful because if the nutrients are missing for depositing calcium inside bone, it should at least be able to leave the body. Oestrogen is given by some doctors to prevent calcium loss *from* bones after menopause but *not* to move it from the bloodstream into bones. This it cannot do.

Oestrogen derived from herbs and foods, on the other hand, can help with the initial symptoms of menopause without any dependence or side effects developing. There is seldom any valid reason for giving prescription hormones to a menopausal woman as they certainly do not behave in the body like her own hormones and have known undesirable side effects. Hot flushes and other menopausal problems respond well to vegetable and herbal sources of oestrogen. Sometimes only a few doses are enough to restore the body's ability to make its own hormones. Herbs containing oestrogen have their effect on the body in one of two ways. In the case of deficiency, the plant oestrogen will function like the human form, but where an excess occurs, plant oestrogen will attach to oestrogen receptors in tissues and prevent the body's excessive levels from functioning. So oestrogen containing herbs can be used in all situations involving hormonal imbalance.

It is only in recent years that women have been routinely put on HRT, whether they have symptoms of menopause or not. If free of the latter, we are told that hormones will prevent ageing, cardiovascular disease, and osteoporosis. This is extremely simplistic, as oestrogen is only a bit player in those conditions. Those who are experiencing unpleasant feelings are persuaded that the only solution is to take hormones - they usually have no idea that there is another way of permanently banishing unwanted symptoms. I am particularly horrified that the women who were experimented on with the contraceptive pill, are now in the same position with HRT. It can take decades for side effects of drugs to become apparent and this has been the case with some aspects of the contraceptive pill. Statistics only now reveal that the sons of mothers who took the 'pill' have a considerably lower sperm count than average and the daughters have a high incidence of precancerous cervical erosions. The latter is occurring at a very tender age - before pregnancies occur. Whilst taking HRT will not affect future generations, it is still a fact that a giant world-wide experiment is being carried out on menopausal women. Another interesting facet of this whole sorry state of affairs is that young women who have a family history of cardiovascular disease are warned against contraceptive hormones, but women in menopause are being told that the same hormones will prevent heart disease. There seems to be a basic lack of respect here for the intelligence of women.

Naturopaths, homeopaths, acupuncturists and herbalists have a great deal of success in treating adverse menopausal symptoms. The key is to use natural methods for relief while the lifestyle is corrected. There is no point in giving hormones when this does nothing to alter the underlying cause of the problem. Sooner or later the hormones have to be discontinued, so surely it is better to follow the decree of nature rather than use toxic means of delaying a normal body process.

Menopause is actually an exciting new phase in life. Usually the children have grown and left home to follow their own destinies and time is available for a whole new range of pursuits. An old career can be rejuvenated, a new one started or other interests tackled. Never view menopause as a time to wind down into retirement from life or, worse still, old age. After all, only half the adult years have been used and a lot more can yet be achieved.

A fifty-year-old woman has directed the affairs of a household, juggled the needs of an entire family, supervised the education of her children, bought and sold houses, designed and decorated interiors as well as gardens and generally done an excellent job of management. She has also nurtured and guided the development of her offspring from the stage of being helpless infants until they are confident and competent adult members of the human race. This is no mean achievement and these skills can be used just as successfully in many other areas. Any fatigue or aged feelings are simply symptoms of an unhealthy physical and emotional body which can definitely be rejuvenated. The same energy we enjoyed in our thirties is available for several decades past mid-life if a healthy lifestyle is followed. You need only the guidance of a natural health practitioner to achieve this desirable state, so go for it ladies.

Menopause is the stage in life when you should be pampering and making time for yourself. In one way you can look on menopausal symptoms as a blessing in disguise. It can be the means of focusing on your own needs for the first time in decades. Instead of feeling low and reaching for HRT, re-evaluate the way you do or do not nurture mind, body and spirit and then use this book to change the areas which have been neglected.

Menopausal symptoms often have an emotional basis. The hot flushes are worse because long-term cumulative stress results in flushes being triggered by small daily stresses which the adrenal glands would normally cope with. The way to reduce this, is to tune into your disturbed emotions and experience them by allowing yourself to consciously feel them without judgment and then let them go. This is the way to shift painful or negative emotions into positive ones.

After feeling the emotion, mentally examine the reason for it, take responsibility for creating it and decide how to deal with it so that that particular issue will not continue to disturb your emotional and therefore your physical body. Valuable insights surface into the conscious mind when you really allow yourself to feel. If we don't consciously experience our painful emotions, we bury them. They are then transformed into physical symptoms and, finally, recognisable disease. Painful emotions have to be transformed by the conscious being if we are to avoid physical stress symptoms. The transformation process may involve allowing tears to flow. This shifts the balance of energy in the body so that the disturbance is freed. However, with the crying, it is also necessary to be clear in your understanding of the problem. Crying with self-pity does not solve the problem, dear reader. However, crying to release the emotion you have consciously unearthed, taken responsibility for and now want to be free of, is very healing.

If your emotion requires a release of anger, then do so where it hurts no one else. Either scream loudly or punch a pillow until you feel the emotion transform into peace. This is the way to stop it from perpetuating your hormone imbalance. If you just express your unhappy experiences on a mental level you are burying the emotion from whence it will surface over and over again until you face it and shift it. Transformation requires taking responsibility, feeling the emotion and staying with it until it transforms into a feeling of light and love, however painful that may be. Often, it is a case of peeling away layers, one at a time until you reach a point where you are able to be free of that particular emotional pain forever; it just depends how deep it is and how long it has been suppressed.

Consider the possibility that your menopausal symptoms are the means by which your inner self is finally forcing you to think about yourself. Tune into your inner guidance system and find out. Those hot flushes can be so intrusive that we are forced to stop and think about ourselves for the first time in decades. If we reach for HRT at this time we are effectively burying the chance to heal our emotional body which may have already been smothered for most of a lifetime.

Take time for you; to reflect on many things, to learn to love yourself, heal yourself, get in touch with your inner power and most of all to feel and understand your spiritual and emotional bodies. In that way your physical and mental bodies will serve you well.

Your intuition is your higher spiritual guidance. The intellect is designed to carry out the wishes of the higher self. Acknowledging this truth at your deepest level, opens up the understanding of your intuitive power and ability to chart your own life pathway. Intuition is never wrong or it would not be intuition!

As a woman and a mother, you may have put others first for two to three decades. Now it is time to stop this pattern - it should never have become established in the first place. Use your beautiful intuitive self (gut feelings) when others look to you to satisfy their needs. Learn to say 'no' if your inner self so counsels and your own being requires attention. Tune into what makes you feel good in life and notice what drains your energy. Be in harmony with what makes your heart joyful. Learn to put a barrier between yourself and those who seek to take your energy. Give love and compassion to them but don't absorb their emotions as that is how your energy is depleted. See the barrier as a pink bubble of love around the person concerned. If you keep this barrier in place, you can give freely without the recipient unconsciously feeling the need to take your energy. When you give love freely, it is always replenished from above. You will not feel drained.

I know when I am not properly tuned in with my patients, because at the end of an appointment I feel very tired if the person with me was in need of energy. I forgot to consciously give and allowed her to unconsciously take. *Conversely, when I give, I am left with an abundance of energy. I am also aware when patients have given* me *an energy boost and I feel great love for them.*

As you heal your emotional self, you heal the planet. As you convert negativity into positive energy, you gain love for yourself and give power to the planet. Conversely, every expressed fear, doubt, negative emotion or action is translated into earth pain. Start by gently allowing your own healing and this will affect your family and close friends. The knock-on effect from your own peace and joy is to bring love, laughter and joy to whole communities and the earth itself.

2. Causes Of Menopausal Problems

When the ovaries stop producing hormones because procreation is no longer desirable, the adrenal glands take over and produce female hormones similar to ovarian ones in just the right amount to keep everything ticking over nicely so that no adverse symptoms are experienced. This is as nature planned. These hormones then travel to the liver where they are converted to recognisable oestrogen and used appropriately. Unfortunately two things commonly inhibit this process: stress which prevents the adrenal glands from doing their job properly, or a poorly functioning liver which does not then have the ability to activate the adrenal sex hormones.

Long-term nutritional deficiencies can affect the function of both the adrenal glands and the liver. A poor quality diet leads eventually to toxic tissues and this too can overwhelm the liver as will pollution of all kinds, be it in the air, water or food chain. In the days when we ate natural organic food because synthetic fertilisers were not available and pesticides therefore not needed, women did not suffer the problems of menopause which many are now encountering. Since we have learnt to eat packaged and processed foods from supermarkets rather than whole natural varieties, all manner of unpleasant conditions have devastated the human race. This has to stop if we are to regain our health and vigour. The human body cannot function properly with a lack of nutrients and one of the side effects is poor female glandular function.

In the majority of women, there is nothing wrong with their ability to make and effectively use their adrenal hormones. The problem is simply that their bodies is a little slow to make the necessary adjustments. Short term menopausal symptoms are completely normal so either be patient or use some of the ideas in this book for relief of those distressing feelings.

In order to reverse *persistent* low levels of hormones in menopause it is necessary to determine the following:

Is your diet nutritionally sound and does it contain foods with natural oestrogen?

Do you have any overt deficiencies of nutrients that require supplementation?

Are your blood, lymph, tissues or any other systems or organs, toxic and therefore in need of cleansing - especially the liver?

Do you have any symptoms of long-term accumulated stress which is affecting the adrenal glands and do you need to examine and free persistently buried emotions which you have not wanted to deal with on a conscious level?

Is your lifestyle in tune with the laws of nature to a large extent?

Is it necessary to add natural treatments to assist the hormone balancing process?

Is it necessary to improve self-worth and self-esteem?

Another interesting facet worth considering, is again related to stress. This can cause premature menopause by directly reducing hormone production by the ovaries. During stress we are designed to not become pregnant so when stress hormones are being produced, progesterone from the ovaries is inhibited and pregnancy cannot then occur. The thyroid also assists in this process. In menopause, progesterone fails two to four years before oestrogen, so dealing with chronic stress earlier could delay the reduction in progesterone levels and therefore the onset of menopause.

What symptoms can I expect?

All manner of events can occur if hormones are not playing their part properly. Here are the usual ones:

Hot flushes and sweats any time of the day or night.

Sleep pattern disturbances either directly as a result of low hormone levels or because of the need to change the sheets often!

Depression, irritability, weepiness, irrational behaviour or being generally difficult to live with.

Fluid retention and dry hair and skin.
Weight gain, stress, incontinence and general flabbiness.
Chronic vaginitis or dry vagina and no interest in sex.
Headaches.
Tingling feelings and heat in the extremities or even a constant feeling of being overheated throughout the body.
Fatigue, trembling, faintness and palpitations.
General aversion to the family.

Plan of action

Check the hormone levels - blood or saliva tests will determine this.
Get a CT bone scan to ascertain whether a focus on bone density is necessary.
Correct the lifestyle in terms of stress, self-esteem, making time for self, exercise and generally following the laws of nature.
Detoxify the system with particular focus on the liver.
Determine food allergies and remove them from the diet as they may be contributing to your hot flushes.
Determine any nutritional deficiencies and replace them.
Clean up your diet so that you are eating whole, natural foods and avoiding stimulants and processed food.
Decide on a natural therapy or mix of therapies to eradicate unpleasant symptoms and correct the hormone balance.
Find an experienced naturopath, medical herbalist, or homoeopath to guide you.

The areas which I will focus on are vitamin and mineral supplements, hormonal herbs, food sources of hormones, homeopathic remedies, flower essences, essential oils for massage, baths and burners.

Living by the law of nature

This involves living in such a manner that the optimum health of the organism is maintained. The fundamental requirements are:

A clean environment externally and internally which means clean air, water and food as well as attention being paid to the function of all the body's elimination channels.

Sunshine and living in a temperature zone for which the body was designed.

Adequate rest, sleep, exercise and attention to personal hygiene.

Wholefoods without additives, eaten in a pleasant environment and to the point of satiety only.

A healthy relaxed state of mind and attitude to life - positive, creative, constructive, joyful, loving and allowing of all things seeming to be different from self.

3. Hormone Replacement Therapy

Taking hormones as a substitute for your own is fraught with danger. Much has been written on this subject in relationship with the contraceptive pill and certain side effects are now widely known. As an example, vitamin E, essential fatty acids (omega 3 and omega 6), magnesium, zinc and the B vitamins are washed out of the system and, as all of these nutrients are important in normal body chemistry (including ovarian function), the long-term effect of such deficiencies may have a serious health impact. Low levels of zinc, B6, magnesium and essential fatty acids trigger depression and studies have indicated that those taking the contraceptive pill during their fertile years, or hormone replacement at menopause, are more likely to commit suicide. HRT appears to prevent the absorption of the minerals it reduces so that when zinc is added to the diet, the body levels do not normalise even after nine weeks of supplementation. Conversely zinc levels normalise very quickly in women who avoid HRT.

The contraceptive pill has always been contraindicated where there is a family history of cardiovascular disease - HRT should carry the same warning since it consists of the same hormones. Studies have shown that oestrogen increases sticky platelets which means that thromboses are more likely. It causes thickening of blood vessel walls and an increased production of the stress hormone cortisol. Taking oestrogen means that the stress response is artificially stimulated on a long-term basis. This is unnatural and dangerous as it wears out the adrenal glands - the very organs needed to produce female hormones in menopause. If we constantly, artificially produce cortisol, blood sugar levels are also distorted because the cortisol blocks insulin secretion and causes the body to make glucose from protein. This may lead to pancreatic and adrenal exhaustion. In lay terms, all of this means being constantly stressed out with a likelihood of developing adult onset diabetes and heart disease.

Cortisole also lowers zinc and raises copper in the body which in turn blocks the fatty acid pathways and increases the risk of osteoporosis. These pathways need to function properly to produce a correct balance of tissue hormones called prostaglandins (PGs). Upset the PG balance and every serious disease in the book becomes possible - cancer, cardiovascular disease, arthritis, multiple sclerosis, etc. PGs control the passage of messages via the nervous system, the health of the heart and blood vessels, hormonal balance, the immune system and the balance of anti- and pro-inflammatory chemicals in the body and therefore a whole range of illnesses like asthma, eczema, arthritis, psoriasis and allergic conditions, to name just a few. The other facet of fatty acid metabolism is that oestrogen raises total cholesterol and triglycerides and may even cause large surges of blood fats. Progesterone exacerbates the insult by lowering the good cholesterol (HDL). This gives LDL cholesterol a licence to damage the walls of blood vessels and so increase the likelihood of heart attacks and strokes. Because oestrogen does not lower HDL, this hormone has been touted as the means of preventing cardiovascular disease. It is patently ridiculous to use such a simplistic reason for taking a hormone that causes so many side effects, one of which is a risk of blood clots leading to strokes or heart attacks.

The stress hormones (increased by oestrogen), known as glucocorticoids, increase catabolism in cells which means that the risk of osteoporosis increases because it interferes with bone cell metabolism. Those same hormones increase blood clotting and thus the flow of blood carrying nutrients into bone is reduced. Alkaline phosphatase (an enzyme) is also reduced which in turn impairs liver function so that the body is less able to deal with carcinogens.

Hormone replacement depresses the natural bacteria in the gut and so increases fungal growth. When this occurs over a long period, the gut walls become porous and the next step is a proliferation of food allergies. Other effects of oestrogen are lowered blood sugar and increased fat storage, fluid retention and cellular oxygen deprivation which is what triggers cancer. Oestrogen also reduces thyroid function, which translates into weight gain because of a slow metabolism. For three decades it has been known that oestrogen thins the hair and skin, so how can this be recommended as an anti-ageing hormone? It is ovarian progesterone which plumps up the skin texture and also improves libido - not oestrogen.

Many women take hormones because they provide instant relief for depression and anxiety and it is true that oestrogen increases happiness. It also powerfully inhibits the ability to learn! Progesterone on the other hand causes depression if in excess. Some women become addicted to their oestrogen dose and in due course need higher and higher levels just to stave off withdrawal symptoms of flushing. Those dreaded hot flushes are usually the result of vascular over-activity triggered by the follicle stimulating hormone when oestrogen levels drop off. In time this quietens down naturally, but for many of us this is not fast enough and we seek a means of relief. However these flushes may also be due to a magnesium, zinc or bioflavonoid deficiency that was previously masked by the body's own hormones.

This book is to be largely about the positive side of dealing with menopause, but I do need to focus briefly on one more important downside of HRT and that is cancer. A recent article in the Journal of Complementary Medicine in the United Kingdom highlighted the fact that top flight researchers are leaving the field of cancer research because they realise that not only are they not slowing the war but they are losing it in a big way. The rate of cancer has increased by 18.6% in men and by 12.4% in women in a comparison between the periods 1970-1975 and 1987-1991. Breast cancer accounts for a high percentage of the increase in women. The link with the increased use of HRT can not be ignored here. Originally women were given only oestrogen as a hormone replacement program but it was soon realised that this gave rise to uterine cancer. Progesterone was then added to the prescription but it is now clear that this drug either alone or when in conjunction with oestrogen, increases the risk of breast cancer. Progesterone is highly immune suppressive which means that our anti-cancer surveillance system does not function properly.

Statistics indicate that the risk of breast cancer is doubled after only two years on HRT. Breast cancer has increased by 32% in the United States since 1982 which coincides with the dramatic rise in

HRT prescriptions. Furthermore, this increase has occurred exclusively in women over 45 years of age. A study which highlighted similar disturbing facts compared women who had never taken HRT with those who had. The risk of breast cancer was 32% greater in those taking oestrogen alone but in the women who also took progesterone there was a 41% higher incidence than in women who never started HRT. Worse still for those who had taken HRT for more than five years, the incidence of breast cancer was 46%. In the women who were over 60 years old by the time they had taken HRT for five years or more, the breast cancer risk had reached 71%. Oestrogen therapy for over 5 years also increased the risk of death from breast cancer by 45%. The good news is that stopping HRT appeared to cancel the risk of cancer, so if you tail off your hormones from today you will join the ranks of women who never started taking them.

I vividly recall an article about a woman who had decided that the only way to solve her menopausal symptoms without increasing her risk of cancer was to find a surgeon willing to remove her uterus so that she could then take oestrogen without increasing her risk of breast cancer. She understood that the progesterone protected her from uterine cancer but increased her chances of malignant breast tumours. Many other women also feel as though they are between a rock and a hard place and so came the birth of this book to show that there are many other solutions to adverse menopausal problems. It just requires patience in sorting out which natural method works best. We are all biochemically individual and so there is no one solution for all women. In the following pages I shall offer detailed help, but it is quicker to have the guidance of a natural therapist who is experienced in using diet, herbs, homeopathy and acupuncture.

Firstly I must put another fallacy to rest concerning HRT and that is that oestrogen prevents osteoporosis. This is at best a half-truth and is definitely not a reason for taking hormones in menopause. In fact, a study reported in the New England Journal of Medicine in 1993, found that it failed to protect against osteoporosis. The study indicated that seven years on oestrogen were needed before bone loss could be reduced and even after ten years there was no protection against bone fractures. Even those women committed to HRT because of unsubstantiated fears, rarely stay on the pill for more than five years.

If you are presently on HRT and wish to stop, this must be done slowly. If you are on a low dose daily pill, spend six months coming off it by stopping one day every month until you are taking only one dose a week by the sixth month. Throughout this time you should be taking the appropriate nutrients and herbs. To stop HRT overnight would shock your body and could cause severe menopausal symptoms.

It is stated in the respected journal "What Doctors Don't Tell You" *(Vol 4, No. 10) - "In our opinion future generations will look back on HRT as the biggest medical bungle of the century."*

4. Osteoporosis

Osteoporosis is a condition where bony tissue is lost, resulting in brittle bones liable to fracture. The word 'osteoporosis' literally means 'porous bone'.

The condition is more common in women than in men although both sexes do lose bone mass. Women can lose 35 to 50% of their bone calcium, whereas men lose 25 to 35%. Bone mass is at peak density at thirty-five years old and loss begins around forty years of age. Unfortunately we lose most from our trabecula bone which predominates in the vertebrae. Therefore women shrink and spontaneous fractures occur very easily. Hip fracture occurs less often but is more disastrous because long-term care is required and often people never walk again without a frame or at least a stick.

The onset of osteoporosis is insidious, without symptoms occurring until the bone loss is well advanced at which stage severe low back pain begins. This is debilitating because of its unrelenting nature. Therefore it is important to be aware of early symptoms of calcium loss in order to take preventative action. These are: cramps in the calves of the legs at night, peeling nails, an increased degree of plaque forming on the teeth or cavities appearing at gum level. Other indications are kidney stones, osteoarthritis or spastic colon. Osteoporosis is not just a condition of calcium deficiency, but more often is due to a lack of other synergistic minerals such as magnesium or silica. Additionally, the bone matrix into which calcium is deposited is normally full of holes in osteoporosis. So treatment is aimed at repairing the bedding for calcium as well as replacing all other elements necessary for strong bones. Taking calcium without supporting minerals is absolutely foolish.

Every day calcium is withdrawn and replaced in bone at the rate of a phenomenal 500 mg. Magnesium remains in place, but this is the mineral that is most likely to be deficient in women because bone levels are heavily reduced after menopause and the food chain is depleted unless organically grown.

The body in general has two distinct phases of building (anabolic phase) and breaking down (catabolic phase). The latter sounds destructive, which it is, but not in a negative sense; e.g. energy production is catabolic. A peak catabolic phase occurs between 4.00 p.m. and 10.00 p.m., and anabolism between 4.00 a.m. and 10.00 a.m. Vitamins and minerals are needed all day long for both cycles, but in the case of bone building (anabolism) which occurs at night, the pertinent supplements are of most use at bedtime. The body is forever tearing down old structures and replacing them with new cells; a wonderful automatic system of continuous servicing. Dr. Emanuel Revici is a world-renowned expert on the subject of anabolic and catabolic phases and has conducted and published a great deal of research in the past 25 years. Upon this research has been built a system of treating illness with individual amino acids because they play a role in the control of these two phases.

Testing for bone calcium levels should be carried out by the use of computed tomography (CT) scan, or dual photon absorptiometry. These determine bone density accurately and the exposure to radiation is low. X-rays are of no value in determining degrees of bone loss.

Hormonal calcium control

Two hormones have a controlling effect over blood calcium; one removes it from bone to the blood and the other deposits calcium in bones. Calcitonin, a hormone secreted by the thyroid gland is the one responsible for calcium deposition in bone. Parathormone from the parathyroid glands situated on either side of the thyroid, are responsible for moving calcium from bone to the bloodstream. The whole system works by a very elegant feedback; when blood calcium drops calcitonin secretion is reduced and parathormone secretion rises to increase the blood level of calcium. In addition, parathormone will tell the kidneys to rescue calcium and put it back into circulation, and will also increase the intestinal absorption of the mineral from food sources.

Vitamin D3

Other hormones are also intimately involved in the process, namely oestrogen and the hormonal type of vitamin D. Vitamin D is important for the absorption of calcium from the gut, but before this happens it goes through several changes in structure. It is either ingested from food or made in the skin by the action of sun on a fatty substance similar to cholesterol. From this stage it is now known as vitamin D3 (cholecalciferol), a hormonal type of vitamin D, and travels to the liver first and then the kidneys. In both places, conversions occur which make the D3 increasingly potent. Osteoporotic people often do not make the final conversion in the kidneys. Reasons for this are still theoretical but the most widely known one is the involvement of oestrogen. However, magnesium and boron are essential to this conversion process and many menopausal women are deficient in these minerals. Giving vitamin D to increase calcium is useless if there is insufficient magnesium to convert it to the active hormonal form.

Any supplementation of straight vitamin D from fish oils in the form of the first conversion, cholecalciferol, should be limited to 400 IU daily because an actual calcium loss occurs at 800 IU daily and it collects in joints and kidneys and as lumps in soft tissue. Conversely, low levels of vitamin D stimulate parathormone to remove bone calcium - hence the importance of the correct dose. If you eat package food from the supermarket, it is likely that your vitamin D exposure is very high as this is one of the nutrients added by a great many food processors to so call 'enrich' the product. In fact these people are a menace as they only succeed in creating imbalance.

Oestrogen

It is theorised that if oestrogen is deficient, as in menopausal women, more calcium is released from bone into the bloodstream than is deposited into bone. Once high blood calcium occurs the hormone system assumes that no more is needed and so vitamin D3 is reduced. However studies indicate that a more likely cause of the high blood calcium is that other minerals such as boron and magnesium are deficient. This scenario will withdraw calcium from bone.

It has been proven that oestrogen replacement therapy only reduces bone loss for a few years, but does *not* increase the levels, so clearly, oestrogen deficiency is only partly responsible for a lack of vitamin D3. In controlled studies it has been already shown that the vitamin D3 is more effective than oestrogen replacement and surprisingly even more effective than oestrogen with D3, so there appears to be little justification for HRT for menopausal women. In addition, it has become clear in hospital studies that although oestrogen can be used to slow the bone loss, once it is stopped the loss rapidly accelerates until it reaches the level it would have been without hormone replacement.

Another justification promulgated for using oestrogen to prevent osteoporosis is that it increases alkaline phosphatase, an enzyme important for bone mineralisation. However, although blood levels rise, the all important bone levels actually drop below the level present before hormone treatment began. This means bone mineralisation is inhibited instead of increased and new bone cannot be made! HRT also causes tiny clots in the blood vessels leading into bone: this prevents the flow of nutrients and is therefore another cause of porous bones.

Calcium

Calcium deficiency in bones may be present in spite of high levels of supplementation. The highest rate of osteoporosis occurs in the United States where more milk is drunk than in most other nations. Pasteurised milk contains damaged calcium and we absorb only about 30% of it. Furthermore, many calcium supplements such as bone meal, calcium lactate and calcium carbonate are poorly absorbed. Calcium carbonate is considered insoluble unless high levels of gastric acid are present. The elderly are often dismally short on hydrochloric acid and have been found to absorb only 4% of the calcium bound to carbonate. Calcium citrate or aspartate absorb best. The citrate form has the added benefit of protecting against kidney stones should an excess be taken.

Stone-age man ate no dairy products and had bigger bones than 20th century humans. Green vegetables, nuts and seeds, seaweeds and fish have high levels of quality calcium and many other foods have moderately good levels. Japanese women who follow a traditional diet, seldom suffer osteoporosis or menopausal problems and yet they do not take dairy products or hormone replacement. A study of their diet is very revealing. Seaweeds, a daily staple, contain very high levels of bio-available minerals and they also alkalise the blood. Meat, which acidifies the blood, is eaten in small amounts so calcium is not removed from the bones to regulate the acid/alkaline balance of the blood. The lack of dairy products also eliminates another source of acidity. Tofu, which is a good source of calcium and oestrogen, is eaten daily throughout life. In fact the daily calcium intake in Japanese women is below 400 mg. Studies are now revealing that if calcium supplementation is lower than required, the body will conserve it better than if normal doses are given. One study showed that even when 2,000 mg of calcium was given daily to menopausal women, bone losses were not reduced. This amount would actually have interfered with every process necessary for preventing the loss as well as interfering with the processes involved in increasing bone mineralisation; an example of the dangers of overdosing on any nutrient. Lots of women self-medicate in this manner, especially in the area of calcium supplementation.

American women who take milk, carbonated drinks and a high protein diet have one of the world's highest rates of osteoporosis. They are only beaten into first place by the Eskimos whose protein/vegetable ratio is completely unbalanced. Their fish diet supplies 2000 mg of calcium daily but the acid forming protein part of this is five times too high. When blood and tissues become too acid, calcium is removed from the bone in order to increase the alkalinity. People with high protein diets are constantly leaching calcium from their bones. The move from normal to low fat milk has exacerbated this process because there is a higher percentage of protein in low fat dairy products and the fats are too low for vitamin D absorption. Moderate amounts of natural, untampered nutrition is a much safer guideline with almost every food.

Magnesium

This mineral should be in balance with calcium. It used to be thought that a ratio of 2 parts calcium to 1 part magnesium was correct, but researchers now opt for an equal ratio. High levels of dairy products or vitamin D (as in processed food) cause magnesium absorption to drop. This causes several chain reactions of events which result in a steady loss of bone calcium. Dr. Guy Abraham, who has done much research in the area of women's hormones, believes that most women overdose on calcium when they are actually deficient in magnesium. He states that a calcium deficiency is much less common.

Any woman taking HRT will also be deficient in magnesium. In a trial run by Dr. Abraham, using magnesium for women taking HRT, the side benefit was an 11% increase in bone density. In those who took HRT alone, there was no such increase. Women are prescribed oestrogen to indirectly reduce calcium loss without realising that this so-called cure causes a further loss of magnesium - what a silly vicious cycle! Even when magnesium is given with the oestrogen, red blood cell levels are only partially corrected. The oestrogen causes a constant loss which supplementation cannot catch up with adequately. Why not instead, supply magnesium on its own to reduce the calcium loss? Because we eat food which is grown in soil that has been artificially fertilised, we all tend to be deficient in magnesium. This mineral is one of the many which is leached from the soil by chemical fertiliser and never replaced.

Phosphorus

Phosphorus and calcium, like calcium and magnesium, must be in balance. Again it used to be thought that the ideal ratio was 2.5

parts phosphorus to 1 part calcium, but now equal parts are accepted as being optimal. Remineralisation of bone has been found to begin only when the ratio is 1 to 1. It does not matter how much calcium is ingested; if the calcium/phosphorus ratio is wrong, bone mineralisation will not occur. Today's diet provides very high levels of phosphorus from sources such as carbonated drinks, processed and packaged foods. Phosphorus is naturally high in meat and grains. Its function is to stimulate the parathyroid glands to *remove* calcium from bone, but it will then stimulate the kidneys to save blood calcium. Calcium on the other hand has the opposite effects. These two minerals work beautifully together as long as they are equally balanced.

Boron

More and more research reveals the broad functions of this trace mineral. It is said to have a regulatory effect on calcium, magnesium and phosphorus, and is found in grapes, peas, green vegetables, pulses, nuts, honey, tomatoes and red peppers. The optimal daily intake is estimated at 2 to 5 mg. Boron activates oestrogen (from the ovaries and adrenal glands) and increases its activity dramatically.

One study indicated that 3 mg daily, doubled blood oestrogen levels and another found that calcium loss was reduced by 40% on a daily dose of 3 mg. One hospital trial discovered that 3 mg daily had the same effect on blood levels of oestrogen as low dose hormone replacement. Surely it makes sense to use a mineral to stimulate the body to produce its own hormones rather than take a substance which causes cancer, cardiovascular disease and depletes vital vitamins and minerals.

Boron is also useful for blocking the damage done by fluoridated water, as it is naturally antagonistic to fluoride. This toxic mineral (fluoride) is still used by some to treat osteoporosis, but it has been clearly shown to cause fragile cortical bone in the long term and is definitely not recommended. Boron is 95% effective in blocking fluoride. Finally it has also been found to reduce urinary loss of calcium by 44% at 3 mg daily.

It is not wise to depend on food sources because fertiliser inhibits the uptake of trace minerals by plants. Things aren't what they seem in the food world any longer unless the food is organically grown.

Bone matrix

This is the ground substance in bone into which minerals can embed. Without a strong matrix, calcium cannot be held in place. Silica cross-links collagen in bone and is also necessary for the deposition of calcium because it is found in new bone but not old. Collagen forms over 90% of bone matrix so this mineral is clearly very important. Nutrients required for the formation of collagen are vitamins C, A, and K, the minerals zinc and copper and some amino acids[1]. It should be noted that collagen synthesis is inhibited by aspirin, anti-inflammatory drugs and cortisone, as well as homocysteine and stress hormones. Flavonoids found in all berry fruits stabilise collagen.

Homocysteine is naturally formed in the body but is normally immediately converted to the amino acids methionine and cysteine in the presence of various co-factors, of which the most important are vitamin B6, folic acid and vitamin B12. Studies have shown that low levels of these B vitamins cause high homocysteine to remain in circulation and that the condition exists in many post-menopausal women. Homocysteine damages blood vessel walls so that cholesterol can then stick to them. Therefore it is vital to not reduce B vitamins and zinc by taking HRT. There is no point in just adding nutrients along with the HRT because, as I pointed out earlier, studies indicate that tissue levels remain low. The hormones in some way prevent the body from absorbing the missing nutrients.

Women with osteoporosis are consistently deficient in zinc and this mineral is always reduced in the body by oestrogen in the

1 Copper at the rate of 3 mg daily has been found to prevent the loss of bone mineral density. It is imprtant for its participation in enzyme activity which strengthens collagen and elastin.

contraceptive pill and HRT. Again it is very difficult to raise the levels to normal as long as oestrogen is continued. Another danger of low zinc, is that this deficiency allows heavy metals like lead and aluminium to accumulate. These toxic substances cause serious illnesses and will even replace calcium in bones. Zinc prevents this from happening but if you're taking HRT, it is almost impossible to increase your levels of this mineral. Vitamin D also requires zinc as a co-factor in order to function properly. Remember that stress will deplete zinc and allow heavy metals a foothold in the body.

Vitamin K is essential for preserving bone levels of calcium and one study showed that it reduces the kidney loss of calcium by 20 to 50%. When the blood flows through the kidneys there is always an exchange of minerals in that whatever is not required is sent to the bladder for excretion, while that which is still required is reabsorbed into the bloodstream. Vitamin K ensures that calcium is rescued when necessary instead of being lost. Vitamin K is also required for the bone matrix in which calcium is embedded.

Excessive salt causes loss of calcium in the kidneys because these two minerals compete for attention. The kidneys recognise the greater need to get rid of the salt rather than choose to conserve the calcium and therefore a high salt diet causes constant calcium losses.

Magnesium deficiency is another reason for the kidneys to let go of calcium as both minerals need to be balanced in the blood. If magnesium is low, the kidneys flush more calcium away.

Hydrochloric acid

Adequate secretion of gastric hydrochloric acid is vital for absorption of minerals and especially calcium. As age creeps up, acid levels decrease and post-menopausal women are likely to produce too little. When hydrochloric acid levels are deficient, indigestion occurs because food cannot be broken down properly. Many people exacerbate the problem by taking antacid powders to further reduce the essential acid. Furthermore these antacids are high in aluminium, which increases bone loss of calcium.

Zinc is essential for the production of all enzymes in the body and for the health of the cells lining the digestive tract. If we reduce this mineral with hormones, we reduce our ability to digest food and extract the nutrients. We also reduce our ability to produce stomach acid and this inhibits calcium absorption.

Essential fatty acids

Omega 3 and omega 6 oils are known to decrease the loss of calcium through the kidney filtration system. They also increase the deposition of calcium in bone.

An interesting study reported in 1995, divided women with osteoporosis into four groups. Each one was given either a placebo (olive oil), evening primrose oil, fish oil or a mixture of fish and evening primrose oils. After sixteen weeks, blood tests showed a decrease of alkaline phosphatase (and therefore increased bone levels) and an increase in osteocalcin in the fish oil group, but especially in the mixed oils group. This indicates that evening primrose oil increases the ability of fish oil to improve bone formation.

Health destroyers

Coffee, alcohol and cigarettes increase bone loss by 50% and a combination of oestrogen therapy plus caffeine causes increased calcium, zinc and magnesium excretion. Smokers have 15 to 30% lower bone density than non-smokers.

A cup of coffee in the morning causes a urinary loss of calcium and magnesium for at least two hours afterwards. The study which highlighted this alarming effect ensured that the women taking part received 600 mg of calcium daily. After being given two doses of 3 mg of caffeine per kilogram of body weight on a single morning, the women recorded a urinary loss of calcium and magnesium which lasted for six hours. The caffeine dose they took was similar to the average amount taken at breakfast and mid-morning.

Salt and sugar interfere with bone mineralisation; salt causes calcium loss by competing with it at the kidney tubule level. Sugar decreases serum levels of vitamin D.

Animal protein

Vegetarians and vegans have a lower incidence of osteoporosis than meat eaters. They have the same bone loss until the age of 50 but from then on, vegetarians lose significantly less than carnivores. It may be that vegetarians eat less protein and therefore have lower phosphorus levels or it may be that because they eat more vegetables their acid levels are lower. A poor acid/alkaline ratio contributes to bone loss by increasing secretion of parathormone. Calcium is then withdrawn from bone in order to alkalise the body fluids. One test showed that raising daily protein from 47 to 142 g doubles urinary calcium loss even when the calcium/phosphorus ratio is not altered.

Vegetarians do need to take care that they do not lose minerals by eating high levels of phytates in grains and beans. These substances claw onto minerals and remove them from the body. Phytates are inhibited by soaking, fermenting and sprouting grains and pulses. Therefore cereals need to be soaked overnight as the Swiss and Austrians do. Rice, millet and barley should also receive this treatment. Pulses are soaked for hours prior to cooking and bread is fermented before it is cooked. It is wise to take zinc supplements separately from food to ensure better absorption.

Stress, DHEA and progesterone

If you have been in a state of chronic stress for sometime, cortisol levels will be high at night and raised above normal in the early morning. This interferes with the re-mineralisation of bones so that osteoporosis becomes more likely. DHEA is an adrenal hormone which reduces the cortisol that is produced at inappropriate times. However it is depleted with age and extended chronic stress so that in time, it cannot reduce cortisol. This means that bone calcium loss intensifies. Studies indicate that DHEA is lower in women with osteoporosis than in those of the same age with normal bone density.

DHEA is also one of the major ovarian hormones and has the ability to convert to oestrogen and testosterone. It may also be capable of increasing progesterone, but indirectly - through a feed-back mechanism. This hormone appears to have the ability to both prevent bone loss and increase bone building. However, using it for treatment could be very risky as long term side effects are unknown.

The important thing is to understand the serious effects of chronic stress and, if this could be a reason for a shrinking bone density, recognise it and treat it. In this way, cotisole levels would return to normal fluctuations and high levels of DHEA would not be required.

For those who already have a bone density so low that they have a high risk of fracture, it may be necessary to use hormones for a short period in order to improve the situation more rapidly. Progesterone is known to increase bone building and this is presently the hormone used for emergency situations. There has been a great deal of debate about natural and synthetic types of this hormone. Progestin is the synthetic type whereas the natural variety is plant derived as diosgenin and then altered to progesterone. The human body cannot change diosgenin to progesterone - it must be done in a laboratory. One of the plant sources is found in the wild yam plant and some believe that progesterone made from this, is recognised by the human body as being the same as its own ovarian hormone. However science has *not* proved this hypothesis and manufacturers are also unable to supply proof. This means that we do not know if it is any safer than the synthetic progesterone. Natural forms of this hormone are already widely used in Europe for treating menstrual problems and are part of some existing HRT medications. There is no proof that these are any safer than the synthetic varieties. DHEA is also synthesised from diosgenin in wild yam and it appears that this too must be done in the laboratory as there is no evidence that the human body can do the job.

I personally advise women with a low bone density to use the supplements mentioned in this chapter and only resort to progesterone if they are in the fracture risk category Even so, you should not self medicate - seek professional help. This replacement hormone is still considered to be a drug and many countries require that it be dispensed by prescription only. For those who are still menstruating, the strategy would be to increase your own production of progesterone with herbs like agnus castus along with supplements.

Diet

Foods to emphasise

Vegetables in abundance, especially green ones. They are high in calcium and potassium, and potassium has the effect of increasing the retention of calcium.
Sea weeds and alfalfa.
Raw nuts and seeds (sunflower, pumpkin and sesame seeds, walnuts), buckwheat and fruit.
Foods high in lactic acid - live plain yoghurt, sour dough bread, sauerkraut.
Wholegrain millet, quinoa, spelt, barley and rice - all soaked, sprouted, fermented or cooked to prevent the natural phytates from depleting minerals. Other grains to be used in moderation and also treated in the same manner.
Pulses - especially soya 2 to 3 times weekly.
Berry fruits such as blueberries, blackberries and cherries.
Foods rich in boron - grapes, apples, pears, green vegetables, pulses, nuts and honey.
Fresh oily fish three times weekly to prevent sticky platelets and calcium loss.
Foods with a high calcium to phosphorus ratio - green vegetables, carrots, turnips, olives, lemon and papaya.
Carrot juice daily, using at least three medium carrots.
500 mg of calcium daily from food.

Reduce

Dairy products as other sources of calcium are preferable.
Meat to twice weekly. Beef has twenty times more phosphorus than calcium.
Salt and sugar.

Avoid

Large meals and overeating.
High protein meals.
Processed and refined foods, carbonated drinks.
Processed oils as they block the function of essential fatty acids in nuts, seeds and oily fish.
White flour and white sugar, and everything made from them.
Aspirin, anti-inflammatory drugs and cortisone.
Caffeine, cigarettes and alcohol as they increase mineral losses.
Aluminium in antacids, aluminium pans and kettles, tap water, deodorants, canned drinks, processed foods and 'table' salt.
Sweet carbonated drinks plus high protein guarantees a rapid bone density loss.

Juices

Green vegetable, alfalfa, comfrey, parsley, red beet, celery, carrots. Pineapple, lemon, papaya.

Calcium foods

1 cup	milk or yoghurt	300 mg
45 g (1.5 oz)	cheese, hard	300 mg
1	egg	30 mg
1 cup low fat cottage cheese		150 mg
1 tbs parmesan cheese		70 mg

Nuts and seeds

1/2 cup of	almonds	160 mg
	hazelnuts, sunflower seeds	140 mg
	brazil and sesame seeds	130 mg
	peanuts, walnuts, pumpkin seeds	30-50 mg

Pulses

1/2 cup of	chick peas, azuki, and pinto	150 mg
	soya - cooked	60 mg
100 g (3.5 oz)	miso	300 mg
	tofu (1 cup = calcium of 1c. of milk)	150 mg
	soya milk	50 mg

Sea Vegetables

100 g (3.5 oz)	Sea vegetables	800-1400 mg
1 tbsp	kelp	150 mg

Molasses

1 tbsp		140 mg

Fish

225 g	shellfish	100 - 200 mg
170 g	herrings	300 mg
28 g	sardines	125 mg
1 cup	canned salmon (pink)	400 mg
1 cup	canned salmon (red)	600 mg
1 cup	canned mackerel	388 mg

Snails

100 g (3.5 oz)		170 mg

Dried fruit

1 cup		50 mg

Fruits are generally very low in calcium.

Vegetables

1 cup of	Beet greens, broccoli, spinach, dandelion greens, kale,okra, collards, mustard greens, parsley, bakchoy, turnip greens.	150-250 mg
1 cup of	rutabaga, chard, cress, leeks, cabbage,brussel sprouts, carrots,	

	celery, endives, cauliflower, turnip, watercress, aubergine, sauerkraut, green beans.	50 - 100 mg

Sources of magnesium

Seeds and nuts		
1/2 cup of	almonds, brazils, cashews, walnuts, hazelnuts, peanuts, sesame seeds.	250 mg
Wholegrains		
100 g (3.5 oz)	Wheatgerm	336 mg
	buckwheat	230 mg
	millet, oatmeal, wholewheats	145-160 mg
	brown rice	88 mg
	rye	75 mg
Fish		
100 g (3.5 oz)	Seafood	40-110 mg
Fruit		
100 g (3.5 oz)	Dried fruit	60-80 mg
	coconut - dry	90 mg
	bananas	40 mg
1/2 cup or 1 piece of	apple, lemon, peaches, mango, boysenberries, melon	15-20 mg
Molasses		
1 tbsp		50 mg
Green vegetables		
100 g (3.5 oz)	beet greens	106 mg
	spinach	90 mg
	Swiss chard	65 mg

	collards	58 mg
	avocado	45 mg
	parsley	40 mg
Snails		
100 g (3.5 oz)		250 mg
Kelp		
1 tbsp		104 mg
Pulses		
100 g (3.5 oz)	soya beans - cooked	90 mg
	tofu	111 mg
	lentils	80 mg
	lima beans	67 mg

Supplements

These will only be necessary if it has been established that your bone density is lower than normal for your age.

- **Calcium citrate** or **aspartate** - 500 to 800 mg daily depending on food intake.
- **Magnesium citrate** or **aspartate** - 500 to 800 mg daily. Take calcium.and magnesium before sleep and separately from zinc.
- **Boron** - 3 to 9 mg daily.
- **Beta carotene** - 6 mg daily if not drinking fresh carrot juice.
- **Vitamin D3 as cholecalciferol** - 400 IU daily.
- **Silica** - 30 to 100 mg daily.
- **Zinc citrate** - 15 mg and copper citrate 2 to 3 mg daily.
- **Manganese** - 10 mg daily as it works hand in glove with zinc.
- **Vitamin C** - 1 g daily.
- **B complex** - 25 to 50 mg daily to include B6, B12 and folic acid.

- **Vitamin K** - 300 to 500 mcg daily.
- **Betaine hydrochloric acid** - if insufficient gastric secretion.
- **GLA as evening primrose or borage oil** - for hormone balance as it significantly increases body oestrogen.
- **Omega 3 oils** - 1 g twice daily as MaxEPA.
- **Strontium** - as the non-radioactive type is added to supplements for osteoporosis because a study indicated that it increased bone density by 78% and reduced pain by 85%.

Any other vitamins taken are to be at moderate levels. Excessive intake of vitamins A, D, E or K actually lead to a calcium loss. If all conditions are optimal 400 mg of calcium daily is sufficient in those who have bone density which is normal for their age.

Herbs

Horsetail, nettles, comfrey, parsley and alfalfa contain calcium and silica. Infuse and drink.

Sources of plant oestrogen are: licorice, true unicorn, false unicorn, black cohosh, fennel, alfalfa and many more. Take 1 g of a herbal mixture, three times daily or infuse as a tea. A tincture dose is 3 to 5 ml three times daily. Sarsaparilla, dong quai and agnus castus are important hormonal regulators.

Exercise

A brisk walk for one hour at least three times weekly. Exercise is vital in encouraging the flow of nutrients into bone and preventing bone loss, but it must be of a weight-bearing type and not swimming. When reaching menopause and we have not been exercising for sometime, we become fat and flabby. As we get older, we lose muscle and gain fat unless we act to prevent this. To remain healthy we need three different types of exercise - the aerobic type is for cardiovascular health, weight-bearing exercise to speed the flow of calcium into bone and weight training to build muscle. If the discipline of regular exercise is difficult, try to find a friend to join a gym with you so it becomes a social occasion rather than a chore.

5. Nutrition

The diet in menopause has to take many things into account. For instance, if you have been in long-term stress you need to pay attention to the recommendations in Part 1, chapter 19. If your bone scan indicates that you are at risk for osteoporosis, look to Part 1, chapter 4 for the relevant diet. If you just need to eat the right food to ensure a comfortable menopause, then concentrate on this chapter.

It is important to eat a good diet from now on as you are eating to prevent ill-health in your mature years. Preventing cardiovascular disease, osteoporosis, cancer and arthritis rests largely in eating in a healthy manner. This means plenty of fresh vegetables and fruit, a daily salad or vegetable juice, only one moderate serving of meat or fish daily and very few dairy products. Saturated fats should be strictly controlled and the unsaturated must be genuinely cold pressed - no margarine, whipped up cooking fats or polyunsaturated oils for cooking. It is safest to use only olive oil in the home. Grains must be whole which means brown rice, wholegrain bread and pasta, oatmeal or muesli rather than processed cereals.

Many foods, like herbs, contain natural hormone-like substances called phyto-oestrogens. These have the ability to increase or decrease body hormones according to requirements. It is important that there is a steady supply of phyto-oestrogens in the diet of menopausal women. Younger people who also do this will save themselves a lot of problems when menopause arrives. The Japanese, with their regular intake of soya products, buckwheat, seaweeds and seeds, do not suffer in menopause and have the world's lowest rate of osteoporosis. One cup of soya beans contains the equivalent of 0.45 mg of oestrogen. One study found that a little more than half a cup of soya beans daily, increased the cells lining the vagina, thereby effectively reducing menopausal dryness. In 1990 another study appeared in the British Medical Journal, again reporting on the effects of phyto-oestrogens in menopause. Twenty-five post menopausal women added the following foods to their diet on a daily basis for six weeks - 10 g soya flour, 10 g red clover seeds which had been sprouted and 25 g flaxseeds. These foods were rotated, with each being consumed for a two week period. This amounted to only 10% of the diet, which is very little compared to other populations like the Japanese who commonly eat half of their diet as oestrogenic foods. The results of the study were quite remarkable in view of this, because vaginal cell quality had improved markedly and this effect lasted for several weeks after the dietary changes were stopped. The other immediately noticeable effect was that the follicular stimulating hormone slowly decreased to pre-menopausal levels over the six week period of the test. This is the hormone which sometimes does not get the message that there are no more ova to release and the ovaries are in retirement. Hence it over stimulates the ovaries and this leads to the hot flushes and sweats. Is this not a simple way of solving hormonal problems in menopause? We truly are what we eat. The beauty of phyto-oestrogens is that the body only uses them if there is a need. Otherwise they remain dormant. In young women who may be producing too much oestrogen, these food types will attach to the hormone receptors in her body and block her own hormones from causing problems.

There is no space in this book to expand on the ideal individualised eating pattern but my book called "You Don't Have To Feel Unwell" has all the information in this area that you could possibly require. The following outline is designed to include foods rich in natural hormones and vitamins needed for hormone production and utilisation.

Diet

Three meals a day - do not skip breakfast. One salad daily to include a wide range of vegetables. Make a dressing from cider vinegar, garlic, French mustard and extra virgin olive oil. One other meal daily is to include a large serving of vegetables much of which should be greens.

Drink a vegetable juice every other day and if your liver needs detoxification, include some dark greens and beetroot in the juice. An early morning lemon juice in hot water also flushes the liver.

Meat or fish only once daily in moderate servings. These should be low in fat.

Include eggs as they are a near perfect form of protein - it is a medical myth that they cause heart disease. Use cheese like a treat and not a daily staple.

Learn to eat tofu and tempeh regularly as they contain natural oestrogen.

Eat other pulses such as red kidney beans, chickpeas, black-eyed peas and lentils. Buy yourself a vegetarian recipe book if you are unfamiliar with ways of making these tasty. There is no need for healthy food to be bland or tasteless. Pulses contain natural precursors to oestrogen.

All grains to be whole and try pastas made of something other than wheat. Buckwheat, spelt, corn or quinoa pastas have wonderful flavours and can be found in health food stores. Eat brown or wild rice in place of the white variety and experiment with grains like millet, barley and corn.

Foods such as grapes, peas, green vegetables, pulses, nuts, honey, tomatoes and red peppers which are rich in boron should be included because this mineral increases oestrogen levels - but the foods should be organic.

Include seaweed in your foods - it can be sprinkled on salad or in soup. Eat good quality calcium foods like salmon, sardines and green vegetables.

Eat unroasted and unsalted nuts and seeds for the natural oils. It is best to sprout them if you live in a suitable climate. In fact pulses that are sprouted have amazing nutritional value. Include sunflower, sesame, pumpkin and flaxseeds, almonds and walnuts.

Eat a variety of oestrogenic foods such as:

soya beans, red kidney beans, chickpeas, and split peas, sprouted and whole grains like oats, corn, barley, rye and millet; pollen, sprouted clover and alfalfa, parsley, celery, carrots, cabbage and potatoes, pumpkin and marrows; sunflower, sesame and flaxseeds; almonds and cashews; bananas, apples, citrus fruit, olives, seaweed, fennel, sage and anise.

Pomegranate seeds contain an oestrone which is identical to human oestrogen, and carrot tops contain a substance that stimulates the release of pituitary hormones involved in regulating all adrenal and ovarian hormones.

If you want to reduce your menopausal symptoms quickly, avoid alcohol, hot drinks, tea and coffee, rich fatty foods, sugar and all processed grains. This means white flour products like cakes, biscuits, waffles, white bread, crumpets, croissants noodles and pasta. Use only whole grain flours for bread and pasta.

Eating heaps of fruit and vegetables as juices, salads or lightly steamed will also reduce the heat in your system. In fact 75% of your diet should consist of these foods. Seeds and pulses, once sprouted, may be counted as part of the 75%.

6. Vitamins And Minerals

Supplements of value

All the supplements listed below have been proven useful in menopause. Clearly, no-one will want to take everything here. In the guide that follows, I give information which may help you decide which to try. The quantities stated are in the ranges used in various scientific studies.

- **Vitamin E** - 800 to 1,200 IU daily.
- **Zinc** - 15 to 30 mg daily separate from calcium. Zinc increases oestrogen production.
- **Boron** - 3 to 9 mg daily.
- **Vitamin A** - 10,000 IU with **vitamin D** - 400 IU daily.
- **Vitamin C** - 1 g three times daily.
- **Calcium** - 1 g with **magnesium** - 500 mg at bedtime.
- **Borage oil** (starflower) - 1 g and **flaxseed oil** - 3 to 6 g daily.
- **Hesperidin** - 500 to 1200 mg daily.
- **Rice bran oil (gamma-oryzanol)** - 100 mg three times daily.
- **B complex** - 50 mg daily.

Vitamin E

This has been studied widely and there is a much evidence of its great benefit in reducing unpleasant menopausal symptoms - especially the hot flushes. It has been found that the requirement for vitamin E can go up by ten to fifty times in menopause. This vitamin is effective against flushes, vaginal dryness, headaches, palpitations, fatigue, nervousness, dizziness and backache in menopause. One study resulted in the total relief of flushes when a group of women were given the following supplements on a daily basis: vitamin C 2.5 g, calcium 1 g and vitamin E 600 IU. The same amount of vitamin E given with Siberian ginseng relieved the night sweats in another study. Most trials with this vitamin indicate improved symptoms in 75% of people and there is the added benefit of moods shifting into positive mode. Vitamin E stimulates oestrogen production and it reduces the overreaction of the follicle stimulating hormone which is a major factor in the hot flushes.

Calcium and magnesium

These days our diets tend to be deficient in magnesium rather than calcium because the chemical fertilisers used for food production leach magnesium from the soil, thus preventing it from reaching the food. However an excess of magnesium inhibits the synthesis and secretion of hormones because it causes competition with calcium for transport vehicles in the body. Magnesium can be taken on an equal footing with calcium and it must be a part of calcium supplementation because the two work hand in hand. In menopause there is sometimes a reduced production of stomach acid which means that certain types of minerals are poorly absorbed. For this reason, calcium and magnesium should be taken in an acid form. This means avoid the lactates and carbonates and buy your minerals bound to citrate, aspartate, succinate, malate or lysinate. Some brands provide a blend of carriers.

Boron

See the chapter on osteoporosis for information on the properties of this mineral.

Vitamin C and hesperidin

Vitamin C is a glandular tonic and it is used as a part of many studies on hormonal imbalance. Taking 1 g three times daily will do nothing but good for a great many health reasons. It combines well with hesperidin which is a bioflavonoid extracted from a variety of fruits. A 1964 study reported that it was more effective in menopause than low dose oestrogen. 1200 mg of hesperidin along with 1 g vitamin C relieved the hot flushes in one study while another one found that 250 to 500 mg hesperidin three times daily with vitamin C had the same effect and this combination also improved leg cramps in those women who were suffering in this manner.

Gamma-oryzanol

This oil extracted from rice bran will reduce hot flushes, joint and muscle pains, headaches, insomnia, nervousness and depression. An interesting study using this product at the rate of 20 mg daily for 38 days was effective in 75% of the menopausal women in reducing hot flushes, sweats, tachycardia, dizziness, insomnia, tinnitus, fluid retention, nausea and constipation. Another study using 300 mg daily for eight weeks improved menopausal symptoms by 85% and had a side benefit of decreasing cholesterol and triglycerides in those with above normal levels. One of my patients takes only this to remain totally free of hot flushes. Some women get no benefit at all. It just depends on the individual requirements. We are all biochemically different and what one person requires is of no use to another. However, at least none of these supplements will harm anyone trying them. Borage and flaxseed oils also control the hormones and will benefit many woman.

B complex vitamins

Vitamin B6 is involved in oestrogen production and PABA will act as a natural substitute for this hormone. Vitamin B5 is an anti-stress vitamin which has an important effect on the adrenal glands. For this reason it may delay the onset of menopause. If any one B vitamin is taken long term, then the whole lot should also be taken because B vitamins work in synergy.

7. Phytotherapy

This term was first introduced by Henri Leclerc in France during this century and is now universally accepted as the term to describe herbal therapy. Herbs may be gentle in action or very powerful. Some are extremely dangerous unless used in appropriate small doses. Those in the powerful grouping often have the active constituents removed to be used in drug form. Belladonna and morphine are examples of this. Most plants used in herbal medicine are classed in the intermediate range in terms of activity and can be taken long-term quite safely.

Herbs contain many active constituents, all with different properties that contribute to the medicinal action as a whole. Thus the potentially powerful effect of one constituent is tempered by other ingredients. It is also a fact that the different active principles act synergistically in increasing the healing effect. For these reasons, the best herbal extracts are those using the whole plant rather than single concentrated ingredients. However, where an ingredient is known to be harmless and highly effective when given alone, it is often extracted and used in herbal tablets, largely to reduce the number of tablets needed for effective treatment. An example of this is silymarin from the milk thistle herb which is used in liver regeneration.

Like foods, many herbs contain phyto-oestrogens which are of great benefit in all hormonal disorders. By attaching to hormone receptors in the body, the plant hormones increase or decrease body hormones according to requirement and can therefore be used in a great variety of situations. In premenstrual syndrome where there is too much oestrogen in the bloodstream, the herbal type will block the body ones and where the symptoms are due to a lack of progesterone, the herbs will cause the ovaries to stimulate the part of the cycle that secretes this hormone. In menopause, phyto-oestrogens reduce the follicle stimulating hormone which is causing the hot flushes and assist the adrenal glands to secrete female hormones. Clever little things, are they not?

Herbal remedies are seldom a quick fix like hormone replacement therapy, but they do work very well given a little patience. In hormonal imbalance, herbs sometimes need to be taken for several months before real benefit is noticed. They must then be continued for about a year to reach a stage of permanent symptom relief. Herbs can safely be taken on a long-term basis for treatment or prevention. Many are used to improve the function of different parts of the body on a long-term basis. For instance, feverfew herb is taken to prevent migraines and arthritis; hawthorn herb improves the circulatory system; and chamomile is a very safe herb used to prevent any inflammatory conditions in the stomach and calm the nervous system. In the same way, phyto-oestrogens in the form of food or herbs can be taken to prevent menopausal symptoms from developing.

Herbs are combined together and dispensed in the form of an infusion, tincture, tablet or capsule. They are blended in such a way that the effect of one herb will improve the function of another or will act synergistically where each has different properties. For this reason you should buy ready-made products or use herbs individually unless you know which ones mix together well. The following are some useful recipes you could happily blend because they are well balanced and of proven value in herbal medicine. Following these is a description of properties of the herbs you will readily find in the stores.

Recipes

2 parts - agnus castus, 1 part each - St. John's wort, life root, oats and black cohosh.

2 parts each - dong quai, agnus castus, black cohosh and oats.

2 parts each - dong quai and agnus castus; 1 part each - licorice root, black cohosh, false unicorn and fennel seed.

2 parts each nettles and sage; 1 part each - mugwort, St. John's wort, and false unicorn. Sage and nettle are folk remedies for hot flushes.

2 parts each - life root, dong quai and St. John's wort; 1 part each - pulsatilla, oats and licorice.
Remember Ginseng, wild yam and licorice if you are stressed, as stress hormones interfere with other hormonal balance.

Chaste berry - Vitex agnus castus

This wonderful female remedy belongs to the verbena family like the herb vervain. It is a Mediterranean tree with sweet smelling lilac flowers. Its common name is chaste berry because it was used in ancient times to subdue sexual desire. Roman women spread these flowers on their beds when their husbands were away fighting.

The great value of this herb lies in its ability to normalise any hormonal imbalance. Whatever is out of kilter will be corrected. Therefore it is used in all types of menstrual disorder, from a complete lack of menses to very painful, heavy ones. The activity of this herb occurs in the pituitary gland where it regulates the follicle stimulating hormone (FSH) and the luteinizing hormone (LH). These are respectively responsible for oestrogen and progesterone production. In PMS, the herb decreases the FSH and prolactin and increases the LH so that the oestrogen is reduced and the progesterone comes on stream properly in the second half of the cycle. It alters the ratio between the two hormones. In menopause, agnus castus stops the FSH from being over-stimulated so that the flushes and sweats can be eliminated. In my practice, I have found this herb to be the single most important one for use in hormonal imbalance. Agnus castus is used for fibrocystic breasts, ovarian cysts, endometriosis, irregular periods, fluid retention, hot flushes and mastitis, to name but a few. Because it shifts the hormone balance towards the progesterone phase, it is also of value in preventing osteoporosis.

Wild yam - Dioscorea villosa

This herb is an adaptogen and therefore useful in stress. Because of its spasmolytic effect, it is used in the treatment of painful periods, threatened miscarriage and ovarian pain. It is also used for PMS, arthritic pains and intestinal colic.

Licorice - Glycyrrhiza glabra

This is primarily an adrenal agent and is therefore of great value in stress. However its adaptogenic properties means that it regulates all hormones. It also contains phyto-oestrogens in the form of isoflavones. Because of the spasmolytic, soothing and anti-inflammatory effects it is used in a wide range of conditions. The anti-inflammatory properties are similar to hydrocortisone and in fact this herb has a direct effect on the adrenal production of all steroid hormones in the body. After treatment levels have been successful, even severe conditions can be prevented from recurring on very low doses of this herb. Very high dosage for a long period of time is not advisable as it leads to potassium loss and fluid retention just as cortisone drugs do. However these effects only occur if 10 to 14 g of the herb is taken daily and this is an enormous amount. I have never seen side effects with moderate doses over long periods. Licorice root is also anti-allergenic, antiviral, antibacterial and stimulates the immune system.

Black cohosh - Cimicifuga racemosa

This American Indian herb is largely used for ovarian and uterine cramping pains. It is also an adaptogen and so normalises hormones. It contains its own oestrogenic substance and is therefore of special value in menopause - in depression it acts directly on the nervous system. Black cohosh is used to reduce hot flushes and fluid retention and in time will even correct prolapses of the bladder and uterus.

Blue cohosh - Caulophyllum thalictroides

Another American Indian herb which may be taken in menopause. Its traditional use is to facilitate birth and ease the pain. It has an anti-spasmodic effect and tones the uterus and fallopian tubes.

Pasque flower - Anemone pulsatilla

This herb increases the regulatory ability of the pituitary gland in hormone imbalances. It is of particular value where nervousness exists because this can upset hormonal balance in menopause.

Rhubarb root - Rheum rhaponticum

The oestrogenic properties of this herb are well documented. It also contains calcium, zinc, magnesium, B3 and B6 - all nutrients of importance in hormonal function. Rhubarb root can be bought as an extract (4 mg) combined with an extract of hops (90 mg) and this product is very effective in reducing menopausal symptoms.

Dong quai - Angelica sinensis

This Asian herb is used in all menstrual problems in China. It reduces uterine cramps, increases the circulation to the area and treats any menstrual irregularity. However it contains no phyto-oestrogens. This herb stabilises the heart, dilates blood vessels and lowers blood pressure and cholesterol. It has immuno-regulating properties and is useful in insomnia and anxiety. In menopause this is one of the herbs which will thicken and replenish the walls of the vagina. Chinese medicine uses it in 'damp-wind' conditions so it is not suitable for 'heaty' people. Nor should it be used by those with fibroids or flooding periods.

Oats - Avena sativa

This has a specific action on the nervous system. It is wonderful for nervous debility, anxiety and exhaustion which is associated with depression. Vervain herb has a similar effect and may be used instead. Take oats as a porridge or a tincture.

Sage - Salvia officinalis

This is a very versatile herb which contains plant hormones and flavonoids. Because of its drying effect it is great for night sweats. Sage will reduce hot flushes, calm the nervous system and lift the spirits in depression. It regulates the sleep pattern and folklore says it stops grey hair and wrinkles. It is also used to relieve cramps and heavy periods. Sage is well known for its antibacterial effect.

False unicorn - Chamaelirium luteum

The root of this herbaceous plant contains phyto-oestrogens and will improve the cyclical function of the ovaries. The American Indians record this as an important gynaecological herb. It is used in all menstrual irregularities and has a reputation for improving fertility and preventing miscarriage. It is a wonderful uterine tonic and hormone adjuster.

Beth root - Trillium erectum

This is the number one remedy for heavy periods and heavy menopausal bleeding which may occur as the hormones are adjusting. It also contains a natural precursor to sex hormones. This herb is used by the American Indians to assist the birthing process.

Motherwort - Leonurus cardiaca

This herb is a tonic for the nervous and cardiovascular system. It warms the heart, comforts the emotions and reduces anxiety. Therefore it is ideal for heart conditions and menopause. It can reduce hot flushes and restore erratic sleeping patterns in a few months. It reduces fluid retention by improving circulation and oxygenation of the tissues, and increases the elasticity and thickness of the vaginal walls thereby improving the moisture levels. Chinese studies indicate that it reduces blood fats and the sticky platelets which lead to thrombosis. This herb is a wonderful link between the heart and circulation, hormones and the nervous system.

Squaw vine - Mitchella repens

This is traditionally used for period pains and in the late stage of pregnancy to tone the uterus for birth. Raspberry leaves are used for the same purpose.

Life root - Senecio aureus

This is especially good for all menopausal symptoms. It is a general tonic which strengthens the hormone system.

St. John's wort - Hypericum perforatum

This herb has an anti-spasmodic effect on the nervous system. It is used for menstrual cramps, bowel cramps and nervous system debility like anxiety, insomnia and depression. It is specific to all the problems of menopause because they also fit the symptoms of general debility. The effect of this herb is restorative. Folk traditions named this plant because of claims that red spots appear on the leaves on the anniversary of the murder of St. John. The plant was thought to have magical powers. St. John's wort also heals wounds and has antiviral properties.

Herbal dosage

It is easier to buy prepared tablets or capsules over the counter and follow the recommended dosage but if you chose to buy the dried or fresh herbs then make them into an infusion. The standard method is to use 30 g (1 oz) of dried or fresh herb to 500 ml of boiling water. Cover the teapot and infuse the liquid for at least fifteen minutes before drinking or storing in the refrigerator. Drink one third three times daily between meals. Where root or bark is used, it will need to be finely chopped and powdered before use or alternatively, roughly chopped and boiled for twenty minutes to extract the properties. Drink only half a cup at a time of this liquid as it will be more concentrated than an infusion. Herbal tinctures may be taken at the rate of one teaspoon twice daily between meals. These and bulk herbs can be bought from specialist herbal suppliers. Whichever recipe you chose from this chapter, mix either tinctures or dried herb in the proportions given and take as instructed in this paragraph.

The following is a list of commonly used herbs for menopause or menstrual problems.

Blessed thistle, black cohosh, licorice, squaw vine, false unicorn, true unicorn, sarsaparilla, parsley, ginger, rhubarb root, red raspberry, black haw, cramp bark, beth root, oats, motherwort, sassafras, dong quai, St. John's wort, pulsatilla, rosemary, agnus castus, sage, mugwort, hops, red clover, anise, fenugreek, fennel, and elderflower.

Dandelion or oatstraw tea will often relieve the symptoms of vaginal dryness.

8. Essential Oils

The sense of smell is one of the most powerful means of communication. In so called primitive societies this is used consciously but our modern society has forgotten the value of this sense for discerning human emotions. However on a subtle level it is still utilised between man and woman. The perfumes secreted by humans are called pheromones and clearly define moods and hormonal cycles. The perfumes in plants are called essential oils. If you crush a leaf or flower in your fingers, the resulting aroma emanates from the essential oil. Some plants produce several types of oil, all with different properties and aromas. Neroli and orange come from the orange flower and peel respectively and are not interchangeable in therapeutic effect.

An odour consists of molecules which are sensed by nerve cells in the nose. These are then transferred to the olfactory area of the brain which evaluates the smell. Aromatics have been used by man since the beginning of civilisation, but it was the Egyptians who were the first to really develop the art of making perfumes and medicinal oils.

Essential oils are made up of many different molecules such as aldehydes, acids, phenols, esters and terpenes: the therapeutic effect is derived from the unique mix with in each plant. Not only can they not be duplicated successfully but, like a wine, the quality differs from place to place, depending on the soil, climate and time of harvesting. Oils from plants grown in their natural habitat are always superior to those grown elsewhere. The many parts of an essential oil act together so that any one ingredient that might be toxic alone is buffered by another. Science has tried to isolate single components, but they are frequently the cause of allergic skin reactions when used in this way. The loveliest perfume in the world is a mix of essential oils in a small amount of carrier oil. Once you become accustomed to using them you will no longer enjoy commercial perfumes. Essential oils for use as a perfume can be blended so that a beautiful odour results; which is also of therapeutic value.

Essential oils have many of the properties of the whole plant from which they were extracted and are chosen according to the healing properties required. Eucalyptus is commonly used for colds, tea tree as an anti-fungal and rose as a wonderful tonic. The quality of commercial oils differs according to the method of extraction and the degree of dilution. Maceration and distillation are the most common methods of extraction; maceration tends to produce the superior end product. There are no bargains with essential oils and you really get what you pay for. The cheaper brands are more heavily diluted and may even be the result of a second distillation of the same plant.

Huge quantities of flowers are required for the distillation of some oils and thus the end product is very costly. Rose, chamomile, violet, jasmine and champaka are examples of this whereas eucalyptus, pine, lavender and cypress contain more abundant supplies of essential oils and so are much more reasonably priced.

How to use essential oil

Oils are best absorbed through the skin from where they reach the bloodstream to be utilised by the body. At the same time they are absorbed through the olfactory centre and by means of chemical messengers, they can indirectly affect all of our hormones - hence the great value in menopause.

In a half-full bath, add 10 to 15 drops in total, of essential oils and immerse yourself for twenty minutes in a relaxed state. When you get out do not rub yourself dry with the towel but dry off naturally.

For a massage oil, add 15 to 20 drops to 30 ml of a carrier oil like avocado or almond. The great value of massage is not only the properties of the essential oils but the healing aspect of touch. Touch is actually an important component of health and should be part of everyone's life. Massage is a way of receiving caring touch which in turn switches on hormones. Other benefits are the stimulation of the circulation and lymphatic systems, detoxification of the tissues, relaxation of tight muscles, pain relief and general stress release. Essential oils can also be inhaled by adding a few drops to very hot water and then leaning over the bowl to inhale the vapour.

The following is a list of essential oils of value in menopause plus a few tried and tested blends. Other useful oils and blends are listed in the chapter on stress and premenstrual syndrome.

- **Frankincense** - is elevating and soothing to the mind and emotions. It is used to eradicate fear and anxiety. It relieves mental exhaustion, burn-out, emotional insecurity and a lack of self-discipline. This oil also preserves a youthful complexion when added to skin care products.
- **Tangerine** - used if a feeling of ageing or emotional emptiness and hopelessness are present. It is for those who live in the past instead of the future.
- **Cypress** - has a sedative effect in burn-out and anxiety. Because of its hormonal effect, this oil increases vaginal secretions and treats incontinence of urine.
- **Fennel** - has an effect on obesity when this is caused by hormonal imbalance.
- **Geranium** - used when feeling unstable, moody and generally depressed. This oil regulates oestrogen.
- **Sage** - normalises hormones, treats night sweats, mental and physical exhaustion.

Blends for specific treatments:

For difficulty in **adjusting to menopause** - ylang ylang, clary sage, orange.

For **resentment** - clary sage, lemon, ylang ylang.

For **lack of self-worth** - juniper, rose, ylang ylang.

For **balancing hormones** - geranium, rosemary, basil.

Aphrodisiac oils - black pepper, cardamom, clary sage, jasmine, rose, sandalwood, ylang ylang, juniper, patchouli, neroli.

Two good **menopausal mixes** are: basil, geranium and bergamot: clary sage, geranium and fennel.

Cellulite

For those who have this unwanted condition it is a good idea to massage the areas daily with a mix of essential oils in a carrier. Two good blends are as follows:

3 parts fennel, 2 parts rosemary and sage and 1 part juniper; and equal parts of cypress, rosemary, lavender, lemon, geranium and juniper.

It is also necessary to clean up the diet, avoid coffee and alcohol and all processed and junk foods. Stress contributes to cellulite as it leads to water retention in the tissues. Kelp tablets, seaweed and silica assist the eradication of this unsightly condition as well as herbs like horse chestnut and hydrocotyle taken internally. Bladderwrack and cola herbs are good for external massage. You need to add these herbs as tinctures to some aloe vera juice and then rub the mix into the skin with a rubber mitt.

9. Flower Essences

Essences of flowers can be used to treat every known emotion and so are very useful in menopause. All over the world people make remedies from flowers and, although some have overlapping properties, there are many unique varieties for which there are no substitutes. Dr. Bach in England was the first person to develop a range of flower essences which he felt at the time were sufficient to treat every human emotion. Since then, our modern lifestyles have given rise to new emotional traumas and so other people have developed flower essences to match these. After listening to a patient for a period, I find a single range of flowers is particularly pertinent to that person and I then focus on them only, but that does not mean that others are not as effective.

Flower essences are made by picking perfect blooms and floating them face down in a bowl of pure spring water. The whole surface area is covered and the bowl left in the sun for several hours. During this time the flower releases its essence into the water. This is then bottled with brandy as a preservative and used as a mother tincture for making the concentrates. Dr. Bach had the ability to put a flower on his tongue and intuitively understand its properties. Thirty years of international usage has confirmed the accuracy of his information. Dr. Bach's remedies are still wonderful emotional healing tools. Many of them are also used successfully for physical ailments.

Dr. Ian White, a naturopath in Australia, has a range of over fifty bushflower essences which he sources very carefully in the wild. He also sells some as ready-made multiple blends. When discovering a new flower he is first intuitively drawn to its habitat and then discerns its properties by sitting in meditation by the tree or bush concerned.

This chapter highlights a few remedies for menopause from the three ranges with which I have practical experience. However it is wise to source the complete sets in health food shops and find the ideal essences for yourself.

Australian bushflower remedies

See Part 1, chapter 19 for useful stress remedies which may not be highlighted here.

Bauhinia - for resistance to change.

Bottle Brush - for feeling overwhelmed by the major life change.

Bush Gardenia - to pep-up a stale relationship.

Dagger Hakea - for bitterness or resentment towards family or close friends.

Five Corners - for low self-esteem and dislike of self.

Silver Princess - if at a crossroads and uncertain of your life's purpose and the direction to follow.

Southern Cross - if you have a victim mentality this remedy helps to understand that you have the power to change your life.

Turkey Bush - if you do not believe in your own creative ability, this remedy will renew your confidence.

Two useful blends are “Confid Essence” and “Dynamis Essence”. Both can be taken simultaneously. Do not worry about taking an inappropriate remedy as it will do no harm. The wrong essence will not resonate with the body energy field and will therefore remain inactive.

Bach flower remedies

See Part 1, chapter 19 for useful stress remedies which may not be repeated here.

Mimulus - for lack of self-confidence through fear. Life is a burden and even frightening.

Scleranthus - Indecisive, erratic and lack of inner poise. Great mental unrest. Fluctuating moods. Quiet people who bear their problems alone.

Gentian - pessimistic about mid-life crisis. Easily discouraged and negative.

Walnut - unable to cope with a new stage in life. Normally knows own mind but now vacillating because of new situation.
Larch - for an inferiority complex about starting a new project in mid-life. Feels hesitant or even useless.

10. Homeopathy

Homeopathy is a natural healing system based on the premise that 'like cures like'. This means that a homeopathic remedy cures the same symptoms in a sick person that are produced in a healthy one who has ingested the substance in its natural state. For instance, the symptoms of arsenic poisoning are the same as are seen in a person suffering from food poisoning and the homeopathic form of arsenic is used to successfully cure this condition. The word homeopathy comes form the Greek 'omeos' meaning 'similar' and 'pathos' meaning 'suffering'.

The history of modern homeopathy begins with Samuel Hahnemann born 1755 in Germany. This brilliant doctor turned away from medicine because it distressed him to see the harm done by blood letting and the indiscriminate use of drugs. During his research he stumbled upon the knowledge that small doses of Peruvian bark were an effective treatment for malaria. (Hippocrates in 400 B.C. had also noted that small doses of herbs were a more effective treatment than large amounts.)

Hahnemann started dosing himself (a healthy subject) with Peruvian bark (from which quinine is derived) and noted that he developed the symptoms characteristic of malaria. This was the beginning of what Hahnemann called 'provings' whereby he dosed people who were mentally and physically healthy with minute doses of substances like belladonna and arsenic and then meticulously noted down all their signs and symptoms. The test subjects had to abstain from all food and behavioural stimulants so that these would not interfere with the symptoms being developed. The resultant provings were then used as symptom pictures to be matched to those of sick people so that 'like would cure like'. The more accurate the matching of the symptom pictures to the symptoms of the sick person, the more profound the cure. This means that substances which cause specific symptoms in the raw state will cure the same symptoms in a sick person when presented in homeopathic form.

Initially Hahnemann treated people with minute doses of the raw substance but found that they often had severe reactions before getting better. For this reason he developed a system of decimal and centesimal dilutions called potencies, whereby the raw substances were successively diluted by a factor of 10 or 100. These were not just diluted but also succussed (violently bashed) so that they gained energy with each dilution. Beyond the twelfth decimal potency, no molecule of the original product was present in the solution and yet Hahnemann found that the higher the dilution the more potent the curative effect. Therefore potentisation removed the drug effect of substances like belladonna but the remedial effect remained. Other examples of this form of treatment are, ipecacuanha which in its raw state causes vomiting and in potency it cures nausea and vomiting; opium when potentised, treats coma; and petroleum, where it causes vertigo, nausea and a spaced out feeling will cure these symptoms when given in homeopathic form. Therefore that which causes symptoms of illness in its raw state will cure those same symptoms in an unhealthy person if given in potency. Any substance can be made into a homeopathic remedy and this healing art uses all manner of animal, mineral and plant life in potentised form.

Today, modern science has an inkling as to why the energy remains and works on living organisms. Sophisticated scan machines indicate a form of memory imprint on the dilute molecules whereby they retain a knowledge of the vibratory energy of the raw substance. This memory is then passed onto the patient's energy field so that it can effect a cure. Two hundred years ago, Hahnemann popularised the theory of a controlling energy field in living organisms, known as the vital force. Today the vitalists even more firmly believe that it is this force which maintains the health of all living organisms and it is this area on which homeopathic remedies have their effect.

An area of homeopathy called constitutional prescribing, seeks to match a remedy to the person as a whole, that is to his emotional, mental and physical state, because it is a fact, that to build health, a person must be treated as a whole and not as a set of isolated components. It is often found that where a remedy matches an individual's personality, the physical symptoms related to that substance also fit many of the health problems to which that person is prone. If this is so, the effect of the remedy will be very great indeed. Where the pertinent constitutional remedy does not cover the present symptoms, it can still be used to strengthen the effect of another remedy chosen for its symptom match alone.

A fundamental belief within natural healing professions is that the mind and body are inexorably linked and if one is affected so will be the other. Therefore in chronic diseases the homeopathic remedy should take account of both. In acute conditions, where the vital force is relatively strong, it is only necessary to match the symptoms with a remedy for a cure and the personality of the patient can be overlooked.

Finally, Hahnemann stated that homeopathy cannot get rid of the cause of disease if it is mechanical or due to poor nutrition. He considered homeopathy to be largely a curative medicine rather than preventative and stressed the importance of living by the laws of nature for the maintenance of health because a toxic body blocks the flow of the vital force.

Homeopathic remedies in hormone imbalance can be directed constitutionally or used to treat symptoms only. I have seen some people experience complete relief from their hot flushes in menopause with a symptomatic remedy used just a few times, but it is always better to match a remedy to the whole person if possible. It is a homeopathic belief that this will create a more lasting cure of any hormonal problem. Matching a remedy to the whole person involves matching the mental, emotional and physical characteristics as far as possible and not just one facet of the being. If you match the personality but the remedy does not also fit the physical symptoms then success will not be great. Deciding on a homeopathic remedy can be frustrating as a seemingly good match sometimes does not work or works only for a short time.

This happened to me. I decided to have myself treated by another homeopath, but every remedy he tried worked only for a few weeks or months. It was very frustrating for us both. Finally I found the correct remedy myself, but not until I recognised certain traits which were a part of me in menopause which had not been a part of me prior to this stage. Sometimes we do not see ourselves as we really are and in this case the remedy fails because it was not in fact a perfect match.

If a particular remedy fits you well, not only will the remedy correct your physical symptoms like hot flushes but it will also improve moods and the outlook on life if this is a feature within you.

Where a remedy is not considered to be a constitutional treatment, use it if the menopausal or PMS symptom picture fits better than a constitutional mentioned in this book.

In the following chapters I have concentrated on the most commonly used constitutional remedies that are specific to menopause and PMS. There are others and some of you may need a homeopath to find a different one for you. Symptomatic remedies for menopause are also in the chapters ahead, but PMS ones are in section two which deals with hormonal imbalances in young people.

Once you have found your remedy, the thorny question of dosage arises. Homeopaths vary widely in their method of dispensing potencies. Some use a single very high potency dose eg. 200C, 1M or 10M. Others go to the opposite end of the scale and recommend frequent dosing of a very low potency (6X or 6C) and then gradually work their way through the higher ones. If you are not absolutely certain that you have the correct remedy it is better to start low and then consider a single high dose if there is a short-lived but effective result. Low potencies (6X, 6C, 30C) are widely available in health food stores but high ones have to be bought from specialist homeopathic stores. You could start by dosing yourself with 6c three times daily for three weeks to see if the remedy is correct. If it seems not to last long this indicates that a higher potency is necessary or that the remedy is not quite right, in which case you should seek the help of a naturopath or homeopath. Homeopathic remedies in higher potencies are dispensed quite differently from drug therapy in that they are never repeated as long as they are still working and the higher the potency the longer the gap between each repeat. In the case of a 200 C potency the gap (if necessary at all) might be three months or more and the 'M' potencies may not be repeated in a year.

In the area of constitutional prescribing, seek the help of a homeopath or naturopath if you run into difficulties or wish to use a high potency.

Homeopathic remedies are dissolved under the tongue and must be taken at least fifteen minutes clear of food and drink. While on this form of treatment, it is wise to avoid peppermint and caffeine.

I am indebted to my friends who provided the homeopathic profiles - do you recognise yourselves? Although I have faithfully reported the symptom profiles of every remedy, they are brought to life as the personality pictures of women who have been dear friends over the past five to ten years.

11. Sepia Woman

The Sepia remedy is made from squid ink. The Sepia woman is one who is seeking liberation from whatever it is that she feels is constricting her. Her physical symptoms have a lot to do with the fact that she has not yet found a way out. It may be her family life which is inhibiting her or her career and she is either still fighting for space to be herself or she has given up and is living in a state of despondency without hope that things can change. The homeopathic treatment will change the mental outlook as well as the physical menopausal symptoms.

A fighting-spirited Sepia woman who is a housewife and mother has a desire to get away from the family so that she can have some space for herself. She feels that she has no energy to give: she feels used by them. However this feeling causes guilt because she has always been a good mother and wife and one level of her being feels obliged to continue as such. Finally resentment takes hold and she may even seriously think about leaving her marriage but her sense of duty and guilt prevents it. Her fear of poverty is also a powerful deterrent. The Sepia mother is not possessive or over protective: in fact she encourages independence in her family. Perhaps this is because she needs her own space. So this poor woman who feels trapped becomes bossy and nagging, and blames others for her own problems. She will become very irritated with people and will sometimes scream at the family in her frustration. Eventually she feels too tired to make an effort with anything or to even go out and enjoy herself. She needs an energy boost to be sociable. All of this may be masked from others as the Sepia woman's sense of duty will be strong enough for her to make a superhuman effort when necessary.

The Sepia career woman has the same bossy streak but it comes out differently in the work place. This lady is intelligent, good at her job and capable of being very objective. She is most often right and objects to having to defer to others or wait for them. Her direct manner sometimes gets her into trouble as she is not slow in pointing out the shortcomings of those around her. She does see her own weak areas although she does not take criticism well, is easily offended and will absorb criticism in a painful rather than a dispassionate way. Her sense of integrity and responsibility in business are well developed. She treats people fairly but keeps herself to herself as she does not like to reveal her emotions. In fact she does not even like to feel her own emotions and will hide from them whenever possible. Sepia women are frequently feminists as they do not like to see women being downtrodden.

The Sepia woman who has either given up or failed to realise that she can change whatever she wishes in her life is heavily into blame and misery. She will sometimes be bossy and fault finding and will even undermine the love of those around her. She is capable of screaming and being spiteful and ruining relationships with her behaviour, but pride prevents her admitting fault. All of this makes her feel very unhappy and so she goes deeper into sadness. She weeps easily, feels intense anxiety and may go through periods where she does not want to get up in the morning, resents the phone or doorbell ringing and feels very stressed. The apathetic Sepia feels no joy, is withdrawn and yet she dreads to be alone. She has much suppressed resentment about past unhappy events and this can lead to irrational bouts of hysteria.

The Sepia woman who has a good job can find herself resenting it, feeling that she wants an easier life like her friends who are not working. If she did stop work, she would soon resent being at home. The key factor is that she is seeking liberation from anything that feels like a trap. By this time, this woman has been a Sepia for a very long time and may even be able to weep all day long and not know why. She often feels exhausted. A Sepia is easily stressed and does not cope with it well. She can go into a martyr pose and won't be helped out of it even though part of her longs to be happy.

The Sepia woman has an inbuilt fear of poverty and this is the root of her problems. This is the trap from which she seeks freedom. She feels stressed unless she can see lifelong security in that she owns a house, has enough to live on comfortably and has a safe retirement mapped out. A husband who does not look after this is in trouble, as the Sepia woman is always looking to others to solve her problems. Taking the remedy will help her to recognise this paralysing emotion and seek help to work through it. Once a Sepia has resolved the poverty trap syndrome, she will no longer be a Sepia in distress: rather a happy Sepia who is in control of her life.

If you recognise the broad outline of this personality, do not discard the validity of the treatment because you do not wish to admit to the negative side. It may be that these emotions are present but as yet, only in a low-grade fashion or they are present from time to time and not constantly. It is still the correct remedy.

An early sign of a developing Sepia is in a young woman who has 'never been the same since' giving birth or having an abortion.

The menopausal symptoms which fit Sepia are hot flushes and sweats which are often accompanied by a tremulous feeling. Her anxiety increases towards the evening. This lady is not much interested in sex, may suffer from vaginal dryness, low backache and restless legs. Her digestion does not work too well as she is inclined to bloating and sometimes gets a sinking feeling in the pit of the stomach. In the morning she may be inclined to nausea after eating. Sepia women often feel a 'ball' sensation internally. This may be in the stomach if digestion is a problem. The constipated Sepia will often experience the 'ball' sensation in the rectum and if this lady has haemorrhoids they may prolapse markedly. Sepia is inclined to gain weight, partly because she eats her way out of misery and partly because her thyroid gland is sluggish. Because she has been stressed for a long time, her adrenal glands are in poor shape and should be treated even if this remedy solves the hot flushes. Sepia is prone to a yellowish skin colour, liver spots in menopause, adult acne and the circulation is slow. Fluid retention is common as is heavy perspiration which is often offensive. The hair roots may be sensitive and the hair falls out excessively. The Sepia woman is unique in that she is cheered by thunderstorms. They act like a rush of adrenalin to jolt her into a better mood.

Women who are born as a Sepia tend to be dark haired, with an olive complexion and dark eyes. However, the woman who becomes a Sepia in adult years, may be fair. After treatment her Sepia traits could well disappear and the underlying constitutional type come back to the surface.

12. Pulsatilla Woman

The pulsatilla remedy is made from the pasque flower. The Pulsatilla woman is delicate with fair skin and a fine complexion. Her disposition is gentle, mild and yielding. She cries easily because her emotions are very close to the surface. A Pulsatilla requires fresh air because hot stuffy atmospheres make her uncomfortable and irritable. However, she also chills easily and reaches for a cover at the slightest draft.

Pulsatilla is largely a woman's remedy because the characteristics are basically feminine. This lady is sweet, gently dependent and always sways in the breeze of life. She is flexible in all things unless pushed too far on a particular issue. A Pulsatilla woman has a sweet smile, her voice is soft, her manner gentle and unobtrusive and she is very sensitive to others. However she also has a core of steel and can always get her own way.

Pulsatilla is the ultimate peacemaker who will preserve harmony at all costs. She recognises the need for tolerance and for give and take in relationships and thus is very fair in her dealings with others. She is never arrogant, demanding or self-righteous. The yielding aspect of this woman means that she moulds herself into that which others require of her. She is malleable and does not have a strong sense of identity. She likes sympathy and to be fussed over and this makes her feel less timid. She absorbs affection like a sponge but does not give it out. She holds no grudges, does not have a mean bone in her body and is penitent when found to be at fault. She is never aggressive or unkind.

Because a Pulsatilla is flexible this also makes her dependent because she actually cannot stand alone. She happily lets others take responsibility for her life and is grateful that they do. This lady believes that there will always be someone around who will be able to help her in any given situation and things normally work out that way. She has a way of creating in others a strong urge to help - probably because of her soft, gentle nature. She brings out compassion in others.

Pulsatilla needs to be loved at all times and this is why she moulds her behaviour to fit the wishes of her parents first and then when she marries, her husband. She is very happy to leave the management of her life entirely in the hands of her husband, but she needs a strong forceful man in her life. He is like a stake preventing her from falling over. In fact there is a selfish streak in a Pulsatilla because she not only yields, but she expects someone else to take care of her. Gracefully accepting affection but not giving it back is another example of the self-absorption. She really does not want to take responsibility for herself at all, not even for making her own decisions. Making even small decisions is extremely difficult for a Pulsatilla, be it deciding which dress to buy or what school her children should attend. She is an optimist but very easily discouraged so she finds it better to rely on someone else to direct her life.

This woman is pleasant to have around as she is naturally sociable, easy to talk to and a good listener. She will quickly respond to a sudden party invitation. In fact she needs to have people around her to lean on. They give her strength. In the evening she really does not like to be alone as she fears the dark and things that go bump in the night. She also needs constant approval from others in order to function well because she is easily discouraged. If she is distressed in any way, crying always brings relief. Life looks much brighter after a little weep. However a Pulsatilla woman is not always sweetness and light; that steel core prevents her from breaking up. Sometimes she will be peevish or even sullen and, if pushed to the limit, will flare up in anger. It is quite a shock to see this in a Pulsatilla because we are so used to the gentle yielding personality.

Sex is important to this woman as she is very sensual and has a high level of sexual desire. She may be promiscuous before marriage but once she has a steady partner her loyalty is absolute. A Pulsatilla woman has sympathy for those close to her but otherwise she does not like to get involved.

She is changeable and contradictory and this is carried into illness where symptoms are forever changing. This is not a classical menopausal remedy, but a Pulsatilla personality suffering in menopause will be helped enormously by taking her own remedy. This is one homeopathic remedy where the chief guiding symptoms should be the personality. The Pulsatilla circulation is very reactive so she flushes in the face easily. For this reason, menopausal flushes create marked redness and sweating in the face. Pulsatilla is very irritated by the internal heat at menopause and is a ready candidate for being easily persuaded to take HRT. The heat is like a sweltering sensation rather than a fire.

Pulsatilla loves sweets but does not do well on rich fatty food. She is prone to digestive upsets with heartburn, dyspepsia, bad breath, flatulence and even loud rumblings in the intestinal tract. She is also intolerant of foods which make her feel hot inside and therefore will pass on the curries as a general rule. Alcohol aggravates any symptoms because it overstimulates the nervous system. The Pulsatilla woman is a morning person and tends to collapse in the evening. Any symptoms are worse after dusk.

A very unbalanced Pulsatilla can become completely inflexible, fanatic, and attracted to cults and dogmas. This may seem like a complete contradiction, but it is just a more extreme way of avoiding decision making. Instead she takes on someone else's belief system to the extent of inflexibility.

13. Lachesis Woman

The main feature of a Lachesis woman is overstimulation: she is constantly seeking an outlet for relief because without it, systems will start to break down. The monthly periods are a major source of outlet for her and many symptoms are better when this flow begins each month. A Lachesis in menopause loses a major source of relief and compensates by becoming garrulous: she will talk the leg off an iron pot! As a younger woman a Lachesis suffers badly from premenstrual tension and heavy periods.

This lady can be mentally exhausting because of her propensity for talking rather than taking part in a conversation. She may pin you down for hours. She is full of creative ideas and her mind works so fast that she will not allow you to interrupt. She does not even finish her own sentences because her mind is racing ahead of her words. She will jump from one topic to another and does not become calm until she has finished. Lachesis holds herself in a very upright posture and fixes others with sharp penetrating eyes when she is holding forth. Her manner is blunt and forthright. In a business conversation there is a brusqueness but this is just part of her fast thought pattern. She is focusing way ahead in her thoughts rather than on the niceties of communication. Suddenly when she has come to a decision she will fix you with her penetrating gaze and go out of her way to solve your problem. This generosity never expects reward.

Lachesis has a split personality and, unfortunately for her, the two parts are constantly fighting each other for dominance. This causes discomfort because the woman is well aware of the conflict. This lady is a kind and generous friend but the dual personality means that you can suddenly be taken by surprise when the opposite side appears. She can become devious and vindictive but because she does not like this side of her personality the conflict shows in her eyes - suddenly she will not hold your gaze. A Lachesis is always trying to suppress her nasty side and this means she is in constant conflict with herself. This woman can swing from being loving to vindictive, from arrogance to touching humility, from being the last of the big spenders to having no interest in buying things, from self-sacrifice to being self-centred and from generous loyalty to deep suspicion and jealousy. Each opposing pole is constantly seeking dominance and because a Lachesis is aware of this, she fears losing control over this inner duel. She is very loyal to her family and will be extremely generous and self-sacrificing, asking absolutely nothing in return. Her feelings are intense and when she befriends someone, she can become quite possessive.

A Lachesis is a very jealous woman - beware the person who gives her husband a sideways glance of appreciation. Jealousy develops because she becomes overly attached to people. This can become suspicion and finally paranoia unless treated. This lady swings between love and hate so one never knows where one is with her. When she 'gets the bit between her teeth' about something she does not like about a person, she will bend your ear for hours on the subject because, although she hates the person, she cannot let go as she is equally fascinated by the very traits which annoy her. A Lachesis woman is also very loyal to her female friends and she will go all out to help one in need and put much time into thought and come up with great ideas. She is actually a very sweet person with great emotional sensitivity who will become teary-eyed when talking about some trauma in the life of a friend or member of her family. However she is not frail like a Pulsatilla; she will do all in her power to assist because she is a fighter.

The duality is most obvious in the area of sexuality and the reproductive system. Sexual activity is a valuable outlet for a Lachesis. (Remember that she is overstimulated in every part of her being and outlets are constantly necessary to prevent meltdown). One persona has a high level of sexual urge, but the other is a moralist who instills guilt and therefore endeavours to suppress it. A Lachesis woman can become lascivious or might completely suppress the sexual urge and suffer for cutting off an avenue of release. The arrival of the menstrual flow is always a great relief for any symptoms whether they are mental or physical because this is an outlet - something is flowing from the body. The menopausal woman uses words in place of a menstrual flow. If she does not do this, or find some other outlet, she may develop illnesses later in life that originate from her inability to relieve her over-stimulation. This woman will say: "I have never been well since starting menopause". This is a Lachesis woman's cry for help.

Lachesis is very critical and like Sepia she cannot accept it in return. When her anger is aroused she is capable of great spitefulness and deliberate insults. She shows no mercy to the subject in question and will methodically cut them down to nothing. The Lachesis remedy is made from snake venom and a Lachesis person can epitomise her remedy to perfection. However, the duality comes into play here as well, because one persona hates this behaviour and will then make amends by trying to explain that the insults were not intentional - that it just happened because some alien force seemed in control. This is actually the truth, but whoever was on the receiving end will have a hard time believing that.

A Lachesis friend is very difficult to cope with because, although she is a very generous and loving friend, she is also shamelessly unreliable. She will make commitments and break them without remorse. In fact she will defend her unkind behaviour vigorously or refuse to discuss it. It is even worse if you try to do business with this person because she may make a firm agreement and then simply become unavailable when it is time to carry out the commitment. This scenario is born out of indecision but instead of calling to say so, she becomes impossible to pin down. This lady can be very devious whilst she proclaims absolute honesty. This again is the dual personality. The dark persona can be an accomplished liar, but the opposing one is never fooled and nor does she admire the dishonesty.

A Lachesis is beguiled by wealthy and influential people and what can be done with money. She enjoys gambling and likes to talk about her influential friends or business associates. However, money is for spending and a Lachesis will do so without restraint. She loves to spend days around the shops on a massive spending spree for clothes and accessories. Lachesis enjoys power, but, if she has succeeded in this area, she will behave with humility and a quiet manner. However if her achievements are not recognised as she deems fit, revenge is planned and she will be vociferous about it to her close friends. She is too full of pride and will defend it to the end.

A Lachesis prefers to leave every thing to the last minute, partly because she works well under pressure, but mostly because she would rather be out and about doing things than settling down to the mundane chores. She is better self-employed as she does not tolerate authority. Her speedy thought processes makes her prone to error; they also creates fatigue. However she is quickly refreshed with a short nap. This lady is a night person who will not willingly appear in the office before 10.00 a.m. and does her best work in the evening. She may even wake up in the morning with an intense feeling of panic.

Her amazing vitality enables her to accomplish much and she is a stimulating person to be with. The opposing side is a Lachesis who is apathetic with slow mental processes. This persona is despondent, has an air of hopelessness about her and will not express her emotions. She is introverted, won't talk and is in great need of her remedy because the shadow side is in control and has completely blocked the other persona. This is what a Lachesis fears most - losing control over the opposing forces. The Lachesis who is still in the driving seat can experience great highs and lows. She is extreme in her vitality as well as in her anxiety, but is not into self-pity. She uses humour as a mask to cover hurt pride and is a master of satire. She is intense, dramatic, assertive, eloquent, passionate and can be utterly exhausting to be with for any length of time. However if she is a friend, you will feel great affection for her in spite of everything.

The prime target for snake venom is the circulatory system so in a Lachesis this is the weak area. She may suffer from hypertension, fluid retention, haemorrhages, a racing heart, varicose veins and haemorrhoids. In fact she can become very anxious about the possibility of developing heart disease and tends to be overly worried about her health in general. She is also prone to throat infections.

Hot flushes in menopause may be accompanied by a tight feeling in the chest and around the throat. They are worse after sleep. Headaches, dizziness and palpitations may also feature. Lachesis dislikes anything tight around the neck or waist and she will constantly pull at a polo neck shirt. Sepia can have this same aversion but she is also averse to sex whereas the Lachesis woman is definitely not.

Starches like bread, cereal and pasta are favourite foods for this homeopathic type and there is also a craving for oysters, alcohol, fresh fruit and coffee. The latter either agrees with or aggravates the system. The grains really mess up her digestive system and often actually cause constipation. A Lachesis will often alternate between binges and dieting. Consequently she is frequently overweight and has a sluggish thyroid. Alcohol makes all her problems worse.

A Lachesis has a real flare for clothes. She is normally beautifully groomed with a stylish hairstyle. Her critical side will bluntly point out others failings in this area, but at the same time she offers advice and constructive help. Lachesis is intuitive and clairvoyant.

A balanced Lachesis manages to control her two persona and will ensure that the modest, kindly one is presented for public viewing. However she is torn inside as she constantly seeks to reconcile her duality. Inner harmony always seems just out of reach.

14. Graphites Woman

Graphites is made from black lead and this typifies the very unbalanced Graphites women. She is heavy and dull in mind, body and spirit. Physically she tends to be fair skinned and dark haired with a tendency to constipation and skin disorders. She is often fat and flabby, tired, cold and sluggish. This lady is timid and has little interest in her work. She fidgets instead of getting on with things and has a decided aversion to mental activity. Her dullness makes her despondent and unable to make decisions. She may spend ages in a plant nursery for instance trying to decide what to buy for her garden but will end up leaving empty-handed because even such a simple thing is impossible to decide. Do not confuse Graphites with Pulsatilla here. Pulsatilla cannot make decisions because she is changeable whereas the Graphites indecision arises out of mental dullness.

It is the blandness of the intellect which is most striking. It is difficult to get through to this woman and she seems slow to receive information. The short-term memory is poor although this lady is quite capable of recalling past events, that is, events which occurred before her Graphites mentality developed. This dullness of mind leads to an absence of thought and by this time she knows that she needs help. Anxiety develops and a fear of impending calamity but there is no fear of insanity.

All Graphites symptoms are worse in the morning - the dull mind, anxiety and the decision-making powers. It may even be difficult to decide what clothes to put on in the morning. By the evening there is a marked improvement. This lady will never be sexually aroused in the morning and in menopause she is definitely off the whole idea anyway.

Graphites' hot flushes are typically confined to the face and she may be inclined to nose bleeds. The menstrual history is of late menses which were scanty. Cutting pains were also typical and constipation occurred at the same time.

This lady dislikes sweets, salt, and meat or fish, with the marked exception of chicken. She prefers cold drinks to hot and may feel nauseous after meals. In fact, her digestive system does not work too well because the dullness of Graphites also has physical manifestations. She may suffer gastralgia, a burning feeling in the stomach, bad breath or sour burps which are difficult to expel. Flatulence is also a feature along with constipation or fetid chronic diarrhoea. The urine too is concentrated and sour. Graphites are prone to unhealthy skin, giving rise to excoriation, persistent dryness, acne, burning or cracking. This is a classical remedy for the early stages of keloids, smelly feet and fungal nails which are deformed, thickened and oozing yellowish fluid.

A balanced Graphites is sensitive, caring, aware of other people's feelings and spontaneous. In the early stages of moving out of balance, these wonderful characteristics become exaggerated so that she is full of anxieties over trifles, overly sensitive and aware, very weepy and feels things far too deeply. Her reactions to events are too intense and she becomes excessively nurturing and compassionate to the degree of being despairing over minor issues. If untreated, this woman eventually becomes dull and unresponsive in mind, body and spirit - probably because the stress of being overreactive is so great that she can no longer cope and shuts down.

In menopause, a Graphites woman can appear to have experienced a complete change of personality. However, her remedy will banish the crippling fears and anxieties so that she is again a free spirit.

15. Sulphur Woman

The circulation is not evenly distributed in this person. For this reason it is a good remedy for menopausal hot flushes where the personality also fits. This lady is warm-blooded and perspires freely anyway. She flushes easily, is prone to red eruptions and burning pains. This remedy, which is made of sublimated sulphur is also good for burning in the soles of the feet at night. Sulphur woman's flushes are worse with heat and especially in bed at night. She may also experience cramps in the calves of the legs at night. Frequent thirst is a feature and cold drinks are desired rather than hot. In middle-age the heatiness increases and she can become more argumentative and belligerent. She may be tall and thin or very overweight. This person loves rich fatty food, meat, spices and junk food. She craves ice-cream, tolerates alcohol well and likes cold fizzy drinks.

Opposite polarities is the main feature of the sulphur personality but there is no fight for supremacy as in Lachesis. This woman can be selfish, stingy and materialistic or very generous without interest in saving. Both of these opposites can be part of the same person. She may swing in and out of the different phases.

A Sulphur is an accumulator. Some save money to the point of stinginess but then the generous side may kick in and the whole lot is given away to a good cause. Then the saving starts again. People who collect swizzle sticks or pens or match boxes for instance may be Sulphurs when they are collecting for the sake of it and not for a purpose. Some collect knowledge and so have a great many degrees or are forever reading informative books. The opposite sort has no interest in worldly goods and makes no effort to save money even for retirement - worldly possessions are seen as a burden.

A Sulphur is a very selfish person, but it does not mean that she is unpleasant because she is normally likeable and sociable. The selfishness takes the form of insensitivity to others. These people are very self-absorbed and do not want to help others. They really don't see why they should and may be quite peevish if asked. The opposite kind of Sulphur is very self-sacrificing because she is over-anxious about family and close friends. Sulphur selfishness also takes the form of being unwilling to lend anything - nor will she throw anything out, even scruffy items of clothing not fit to be seen in public.

A Sulphur is either very interested in clothes or totally unaware. However, even if she is beautifully dressed, there will often be a dirty mark somewhere or a shoe is scuffed - something spoils the perfect image. Sulphurs are not very keen on washing and they can be very dirty in the home - especially the bathroom. The wash basin is not cleaned after use and toothpaste is frequently just left oozing from the tube on the side of the basin. The opposite Sulphur type, by contrast, will shower several times a day. A Sulphur cannot tolerate odours and will be big into air fresheners and making sure no cooking smells reach the living room. She hates waste and will make petty economies even when money is no object.

A Sulphur can be very untidy, but not usually both at work and home. One place is likely to be neat but not the other. This woman is either intellectual with an inquiring mind or averse to mental exertion and muddle headed. One type of Sulphur has a very high self-esteem and needs recognition of her talents. She will argue vigorously to show how clever she is and may be very boastful. The opposite type has no interest in intellectual pursuits, no hang-ups, is very hospitable, happy and enjoys life. Neither type cares a hoot about what others think.

This remedy is very deep acting and will often bring latent symptoms to the surface. However it often has no effect whatever on Sulphur's annoying personality traits.

16. Kali Carb. Woman

This remedy is made from potassium carbonate and the Kali carb. woman has an inflexible sense of duty and right and wrong. Everything is seen in terms of black and white only. She is uptight and, although she is sensitive underneath the mask, you would never know it. Kali carb. keeps an iron control over her emotions. For this reason she has no means of releasing problems externally whether they are mental or emotional. Hence her physical body absorbs the stresses and can reach a stage where structures are deformed. Kali carb. is a major remedy for arthritis where the joints are twisted out of shape. Emotions such as anxiety and fear are frequently felt as a pain in the stomach. They do not register in the mind of this rigid, dogmatic woman.

Because this lady is so controlled, her symptoms are always worse when there is the least resistance - that is, at 2.00 to 4.00 a.m., when the body is at its lowest ebb. Menopausal hot flushes and sweats will occur within this time frame. In the extreme, this lady cannot sleep, simply because she cannot let go of control in order to relax.

A Kali carb. woman may refuse to even acknowledge her hormonal imbalance and as the symptoms worsen she becomes very irritated because her body is not functioning correctly. However this will still not encourage her to seek help and neither will she complain because that would require accepting that she has a problem. If you recognise yourself here, please seek help or otherwise the situation will worsen until it may be too late for a complete cure of your problems. In spite of the fact that this woman will appear to have no interest in another person's traumas, she is in fact quite sensitive, but does not show it. She will quietly mull over the issue and come up with a solution.

This woman has a strong desire for sweets, but coffee makes her feel unwell. She does not like to be alone and is very afraid of the dark. The slightest draft is intensely annoying to a Kali carb. and will not be tolerated.

17. Folliculinum Woman

This remedy is made from a synthetic oestrogen and was developed in the 1940's by Dr. Donald Foubister, a medical doctor who became an expert in homeopathy. His work on remedies for surgical cases is without precedent. In 1960 Dr. Foubister became Dean of the Faculty of Homeopathy at the Royal London Homeopathic Hospital and was a consultant physician there. Eventually he was elected president of the faculty in recognition of his enormous contribution to this healing art.

The guiding symptom for this remedy is of a person full of self denial who loses herself in relationships. She tends to be a doormat who has not developed a personality of her own. This is because of a depressed unhappy childhood. She probably had very strict parents who prevented her from developing in her own way. She may even have been beaten or abused. This child probably had difficulty standing up to bullies at school and was unduly anxious about exams. This arises where the parents are more interested in the scholastic achievements than in the child as a person.

Because this woman was not allowed to be herself as a child, in adulthood she is unsure of herself, easily hurt or upset and does not like to be alone. She often feels as though others are feeding off her emotionally or that she is controlled by them. This leads to aggressive feelings which fold into depression.

A Folliculinum woman who had a strict upbringing may be into self-imposed control. She did this as a child to avoid trouble and is still doing it as an adult. This may be so extreme that she will even give up the chance of a happy marriage in order to devote years to nursing aged parents. This lady is out of sorts with all her body rhythms - especially the hormonal ones. She may even suffer eating disorders which are a form of self-abuse.

This is a wonderful remedy for PMS and all menopausal symptoms. However it is not a major constitutional remedy. Dr. Foubister recommended giving folliculinum 30C for three to four days before the constitutional remedy. Sepia is the usual one to follow Folliculinum because a Sepia woman also suffers emotional insecurity, feels controlled by others and is easily hurt and upset. However, for some women in menopause, a few doses of folliculinum alone will banish menopausal symptoms forever.

This remedy is also appropriate for a teenaged girl who is drained, slow and unable to identify 'self', especially if her mother took the contraceptive pill prior to conception. It may help in infertility and where menses have become irregular since stopping the pill.

18. Other Homeopathic Remedies

Some menopausal women do very well using homeopathic oestrogen for the period their bodies are taking to adjust to the altered hormone balance. Remember that those annoying symptoms are normal. The reason that you are experiencing discomfort is that your body is slow to adjust to the changes and therefore life is made easier by using something natural to bring relief whilst you wait. Don't suppress the symptoms with drug forms of hormone treatment as that is not helping the body to adjust to the hormonal change; it is replacing your own natural ones with a type which carries serious health risks and prevents menopause from occurring. Hormones usually adjust fairly quickly but, if not, you must look to treating your accumulated and ongoing stress as this is possibly preventing the female hormones from flowing from the adrenal glands as nature intended.

If a preceding constitutional remedies did not fit, try one of the following. These remedies are very good in menopause if the symptom patterns fit your particular type of flushes and moods. Buy the 6C potency of the appropriate remedy and take it three times daily until the problems are relieved.

Sulphuric acidum

For hot flushes which are followed by perspiration with a weak trembling sensation. The symptoms are worse in the upper part of the body and worse in the evening, particularly after exercise. Great weariness is a feature of this remedy. The smell of coffee is nauseating, but this person craves alcohol and has a desire for fresh food. She is fretful, impatient, always in a hurry and unwilling to talk about her symptoms.

Crolatus

For women with a menstrual history of pain extending down the thighs during menses and a feeling of the uterus about to fall out. The hot flushes may manifest as itchy bumps which appear in specific areas of the body. The legs are forever moving or she feels uncomfortable.

Amyl nitrate

This remedy acts on the capillaries which is why it is so suitable in menopause. The hot flushes result from instability of these tiny blood vessels. This remedy works where the flushes are powerfully overwhelming and have a very sudden onset. The main area affected is the face and head region and the flush is followed by sweating. This woman may have a sensation of tumultuous head activity. She is prone to headaches, anxiety and palpitations.

Sanguinaria

This is a remedy for hot flushes that are felt mostly in the head and chest area. The palms of the hands and soles of the feet may also burn intensely and the cheeks burn a bright red colour. Headaches may be a part of menopause and pain in the shoulder is one of the distinctive unusual features. This woman has a history of heavy profuse periods.

Kreosotum

This woman's hot flushes occur as a real burning heat and night sweats are also a feature. There is a menstrual history of menses ceasing when walking or sitting, then reappearing when lying down. This remedy also covers irritability, peevishness and forgetfulness.

Veratrum viride

A remedy for flushes that are like overwhelming rushes to the head which cause great prostration. Rapid congestion is the guiding indication. This fits women who are inclined to be of high colour normally or even quite livid. They are also quarrelsome types.

Glonoinum

This will help those who suffer sudden, violent and unexpected flushes. There is a feeling of brain congestion because of the surge of blood to the head and the heart. The skull feels as though there is not enough space for the brain. There is a pulsating feeling throughout the body and throbbing in the head. Sometimes there are waves of heat moving upwards from the pit of the stomach. This may be accompanied by nausea which is relieved by the perspiration. This lady is extremely irritable and lethargic and may feel dizzy on standing up. Symptoms are worse in the morning and with exertion of any kind. The sun worsens her problems and she really suffers a hot climate.

Jab

Recommended for when flushes are accompanied by sudden excessive perspiration. There is a feeling of heat with throbbing. The face goes red and then quite pale.

Cimicifuga

This is for hot flushes accompanied by a weak sinking feeling in the pit of the stomach. Headaches occur and there is irritability, restlessness and depression that feels like being enveloped in a cloud.

19. Stress

Stress is defined as anything that threatens the health of the body or has an adverse effect on its functioning, such as injury, disease, depression or worry. The presence of one form of stress diminishes resistance to other types. For instance when a person is ill he cannot cope adequately with worry and will notice that minor upsets are blown out of proportion. Constant stress brings about hormonal changes in the body and also reduces the thyroid and immune function sleep quality, bone density, skin regeneration, muscle and joint function.

Stress in moderation is the spice of life and we would be very dull people without it. A certain level acts as incentive in every aspect of our lives and as such is important to our survival. So positive stress is not harmful and is indeed necessary. What is important is the response to it. If a heavy work load is viewed as a burden then stress is present. On the other hand, if it is viewed as a challenge or even a pleasure, then stress does not occur. The response depends on the type of person. An 'A' type who is constantly on the move, drives herself hard, sets impossible deadlines, is ambitious and can't relax will accumulate stress rapidly. A 'B' type person who is much more laid back in every way will not, although she may also be ambitious. What is a major stress to an 'A' type person is of no importance to a 'B' type and an example of this is when considering meeting impossible deadlines. The person who does not respond correctly to the stress will panic over being late whereas the person who does react adequately will accept the impossibility with equanimity and just do her best to finish as soon as possible. Clearly everyone should endeavour to become more relaxed about life in order to prevent stress induced illness.

Alternatively, where potential stress loads cannot be reduced, it is important to react differently so that tension is released instead of internalised. When anger is aroused over trifles, stop and examine the problem and deliberately put it in perspective. If the anger is due to a major event, be sure to remove it harmlessly by expressing your feelings appropriately or using a deep breathing exercise or relaxation technique. For some, a primordial scream may be appropriate.

Stress is cumulative and we become less able to cope with its symptoms as time passes. Unless an adequate response is mounted every time, physical illness or hormone imbalance will eventually occur. For this reason it is important to also avoid the pitfall of no response, as stresses buried inside are as harmful as an uncontrolled flaring anger, anxiety or depression over small events. When unhappiness, anxiety, jealousy, fear or rejection is buried, it festers and becomes internal hostility or anger which is harmful. Feelings must be expressed and solutions found to these painful emotional events. Once the load has become heavy, a single minor event may tip the balance from adaptation to stress into physical illness.

It is important to accept that we have free choice as to how we react to events, people and emotions, because only then is it possible to make the necessary changes in attitudes, responses, personality and pace of life. The people who cope well with stress are not only the 'B' types. Those who are somewhere in the middle, but have what is known as a hardiness factor, also respond well. They have control over all aspects of their lives which means that they, rather than others, determine their thoughts and actions. Outside influences are only secondary. These people have an inner sense of responsibility and know they can chart their own course. Outside influences are only secondary.

Those who feel at the mercy of others, who don't make their own decisions and blame someone else for life's misfortunes have a very low hardiness level. Viewing life as a challenge and seeing it as something exciting also increases hardiness as does feeling involved in life in general. By this, I mean being stimulated by events, people, places and situations outside one's immediate environment. Parents can do much to encourage these healthy traits in their offspring but even adults can learn with the help of counselling and supportive friends. Just becoming aware of the need for change and accepting its possibility is a major step on the road to becoming a well person.

The causes of stress

There is an endless list of things which have the potential for causing stress and it is interesting to note that even happy events can be perceived as stressful. A rating system for lifestyle changes was developed by the researchers Holmes and Lake in the 1960's whereby stressful events were allocated specific numbers according to the degree of harm they could cause. Death of a spouse has the highest score of 100 while divorce rates 73. A happy event like marriage is more stressful than losing a job or retiring and pregnancy is rated the same as sex problems. In fact, anticipating changes in lifestyle is actually worse in terms of stress than dealing with the reality. For instance, the fear of losing a job is worse than finding a new one.

Dangerous jobs are stressful. The police and firemen have high stress levels and men who have to climb dangerous scaffoldings for a living, pump out lots of stress hormones. Being caught in a traffic jam without a phone in the car is a problem to many as the thought of being late is stressful. Emotions such as guilt, resentment, self-pity, self-loathing, anger, depression, anxiety or brooding over conflicts are all causes of cumulative stress unless they are harmlessly discharged. An inability to defuse emotions by talking them through is very harmful. An adequate response returns everything to normal. In the face of a charging bull it is normal to run, but an adequate response to anger is a calm evaluation, to discuss it or free it by some other method.

Chronic stress symptoms

When acute reactions to stress become chronic, muscles remain tense in some areas and anxiety may become constant. Hormones remain altered and the adrenal glands conserve sodium to maintain a normal blood pressure. Infections become chronic or occur frequently because of the constantly lowered immune response and wound healing becomes slow.

Blood sugar disturbances may become a regular feature because sugar and fats are being continually broken down for the energy that is required to meet the emotional crisis. This means that blood sugar levels see-saw, causing periodic sugar craving, irritability, weepiness, headaches and even the shakes. The insulin response to sugar surges damages blood vessels, as do the stress hormones. Other symptoms of being in chronic stress are:

Constant fatigue and disturbed sleep patterns. Those who cannot go to sleep easily or who wake and do not go back to sleep are stressed. When cortisol is high at night (in chronic stress), bone re-building is seriously compromised over an extended period. This could lead to osteoporosis.

Thyroid dysfunction with resultant changes in metabolism.

Poor wound healing and skin regeneration.

Eating disorders; either over-indulgence or a loss of appetite. Some people will even turn away from a previously healthy diet and start routinely reaching for the worst kinds of junk food when stressed.

Nervous disorders like nail-biting, being unable to sit still and relax, twitching muscles, a tight chest, headaches and palpitations.

When the nervous system control of organs goes awry, excessive sweating, irritable bowel syndrome, constipation or diarrhoea may occur. Cystitis or urethritis are frequently caused by stress rather than an infecting organism.

Emotional disturbances such as suppressed anger or crying too easily, feeling unloved, misunderstood, being fearful and anxious, a lack of self esteem, irritability out of proportion to the event and a feeling that things frequently go wrong.

Being unable to plan or follow a schedule for coping with the workload.

Not making time for self and worrying about the future.

Unexplained pains occurring anywhere in the abdomen or chest.

Development of allergies or an auto-immune disease, whereby the body destroys its own tissue. Frequent infections and an unhealthy intestinal environment are also due to immune system damage from stress hormones.

Menopausal symptoms of all kinds, including a low sex drive or periodic hot flushes, feeling uncomfortable or irritable about touching or being touched, extreme mental or physical lethargy and volatile emotions.

If you have been stressed over a long period in the past, it is important to realise that even seemingly minor stressful situations in the present will affect your adrenal glands very strongly. This means that female hormones will cease to be secreted when, once again, the adrenals focus on putting out stress hormones. The effect of stress on the adrenals is cumulative and eventually they become too tired to secrete female hormones at the same time as coping with making stress hormones. Self-preservation dictates that the glands prioritise. If you are in this situation, it will be vital for you to markedly increase your intake of oestrogenic foods. For some, it may even be necessary to use an oestrogen cream in minute amounts for a few weeks while the stressful situation is dealt with. Then, long-term changes in lifestyle *are vital for the adrenals to recover to the extent that occasional serious stress does not halt the flow of oestrogen.*

Diet

Someone who is stressed has a major need for an increased amount of vitamins, minerals and enzymes. To this end, everything that is eaten should be of top quality in terms of nutritional value. Many people think that eating processed food is all right because it won't actually do any harm. However, if you eat a bowl of processed cereal (which is not much better than a bowl of sugar), you will be full without ever having a food rich in nutrients and the body will have to wait another few hours in the hope of receiving good food.

Follow the PMS or menopausal diet in this book and make sure that 65% of the food is raw in the form of fruit, vegetables, seeds, nuts and cereals. Remember that raw cereals should be soaked, sprouted or fermented, so that minerals are not leached from the body. If you are in menopause, also ensure that oestrogen foods are part of your regime. (See menopausal diet)

Make real efforts to avoid white flour and all sugar and everything made from them. This means avoiding bread that is even partially made from white flour, pizza, pasta, cakes, crumpets, pancakes and pastry. Avoid jams, soft drinks, squashes, tea, coffee and the many cocoa type drinks. Everything eaten should be made from natural fresh food and not come from packets, cans or the freezer section of the supermarket. Sweet treats can be made from wholewheat flour with honey or maple syrup used in place of sugar. Buy brown rice instead of white, muesli or porridge oats, instead of pretty packaged cereals, whole grain flour and make your own cakes, pizzas and pancakes. Wholewheat, cornmeal, quinoa and buckwheat pastas are widely available. I never understand someone choosing the white variety when the wholegrain has the enormous advantage or never going sticky. Some brands taste better than others, so experiment. Change from crisps and processed snacks to eating raw fresh nuts, olives, crudities and home made dips, such as hommous and live yoghurt based varieties. In restaurants choose salad with beans or cottage cheese, eggs and an olive oil/lemon juice dressing. Skip the white pasta and potato salad covered in thick poor quality mayonnaise and definitely skip the croutons. Choose fresh fish with a variety of vegetables and a side salad and ask for wholewheat bread when the white rolls arrive. Freshly made soups make good starters and fresh fruit or cheese and wholewheat bread/crackers can finish a meal. A glass of wine with the evening meal is permissible but drink a mineral water with a squeeze of lemon otherwise. Herbal teas can replace tea and coffee and dandelion and barley grain 'coffees' are available.

Treatments of value

Bach flowers

These essences taken to rebalance whichever emotions are out of control can help stressed people enormously. Some of the useful ones are detailed below, but there are thirty-eight flower remedies and a stressed person would be wise to read up on this and choose up to any five which are the most appropriate.

Impatiens - is for the impatient person who is always in a hurry and would rather do something himself than take the time to teach another. These people react quickly, are irritable, difficult to please, nervy, intolerant of restraint and restless. They don't tolerate fools and cannot wait for events to take their course.

White chestnut - is for those who cannot put aside problems. They prey on the mind and even prevent sleep. This essence is for mental tension, teeth grinding, chronic headaches, fatigue and depression. It is also for those people who have constantly whirring minds which cause great mental and physical tension.

Olive - is for complete physical and mental exhaustion after a long period of strain. This person feels washed out without reserves and everything is an effort.

Heather - is for the self-centred person who has reached the stage of making mountains out of molehills, weeps easily, and is full of self-pity.

Elm - is for those who feel temporarily overwhelmed by responsibility. These people are normally very capable.

Australian bushflower remedies

Crowea - is for those who constantly worry or experience anxiety. It is also appropriate for that 'not quite right' feeling; for those who always worry about something, but never have specific fears. It is also good for worriers with stomach upsets.

Bottle brush - The remedy brings calm and the ability to cope during major life changes which are stressful.

Banksia robur - is for the weary, disheartened, frustrated person who is low in energy. This remedy is for those who are normally very dynamic but are temporarily burnt out.

Paw paw - is for feeling overwhelmed with problems and burdened by the decisions which have to be made. It brings calmness and clarity of mind and goes well with crowea.

Macrocarpa - has an affinity for the adrenal glands. It is for exhaustion and burn-out and acts as a pick-me-up.

Ian White has developed fifty Australian flower remedies and, although some overlap with Dr. Edward Bach's flowers, many are unique and useful for the problems we face in modern life.

Nutrients to support the adrenal glands

- **Vitamin B complex** - 50 mg daily or Brewer's yeast, 1 to 2 tablespoons daily.
- **Vitamin B5 (Pantothenic acid)** - 500 mg daily.
- **Vitamin B3 (niacinamide)** - 0.5 to 3 g daily.
- **Vitamin C** - 1 g twice daily.
- **Beta carotene** - 6 mg daily.
- **Vitamin E** - 200 IU daily.
- **Selenium** - 200 mcg daily.
- **Zinc** - 25 mg daily.
- **Manganese** - 5 to 10 mg daily.
- **Kelp** tablets for natural sodium and other minerals.

An immune stimulating formulation contains many of the above in similar dosage. Some people may need higher doses of the vitamins B3, B6 and B5. Dr. A. Hoffer, the international authority on vitamin B3, recommends that people who are stressed take the high dose as it is the specific antidote to the harmful effects of adrenalin. He also advises that they routinely take adequate amounts of the anti-oxidants, vitamins A, C, E and selenium. Vitamin B3 is very effective in anxiety states, when floods of adrenalin are produced, but it is not generally called for in chronic stress. Only take high doses if it is prescribed.

- **Calcium** and **magnesium** - 400 to 800 mg daily of each as citrate, aspartate or amino acid chelate.
- **Inositol** - 250 mg three times daily of this B vitamin has an anti-anxiety effect on brain waves (similar to Valium).
- **GABA** - an amino acid very useful for aborting panic attacks or for chronic anxiety. Dissolve 300 mg under the tongue as necessary. It is also useful for inducing sleep.
- **Glutamic acid** - 250 mg three times daily. It is another amino acid which calms the brain waves in anxiety.
- **L-tyrosine** - 500 mg twice daily for the formation of adrenalin and to regulate emotions and moods.
- **L-histidine** - 500 mg three times daily is an amino acid for calming the mind of anxious people.

Herbs

These are to strengthen the adrenal glands.

- **Ginseng** - 1 to 2 g three times daily for tuning the adrenal cortex to respond correctly to stress. It is a very potent adaptogen which balances the adrenal hormones as well as oestrogen and progesterone. The thyroid and pituitary functions are also regulated.
- **Licorice root** - 400 mg three times daily reacts with the part of the adrenal gland controlling sodium and fluid levels and reduces stress damage to the adrenal cortex. It affects potassium balance in long term usage but only in much higher doses.
- **Wild yam** - 1 g three times daily for its relaxant and adaptogenic properties
- **Chinese thoroughwax** - 2 to 4 g three times daily increases adrenal hormones and enhances their effect.

The Brazilian herbs guarama and suma also support adrenal function.

In chronic stress, herbal doses are generally low as high levels may overstimulate tired adrenal glands. The aim of treatment is to support natural function.

Herbs

These are for the nervous system - take three times daily:

- **Passiflora** - 0.25 to 1 g dried herb for insomnia and anxiety.
- **Betony** - 2 to 4 g dried herb for stress, anxiety and tension headaches.
- **Valerian** - 0.03 to 1 g dried herb improves sleep latency. However in some people this herb does not degrade properly and acts as a stimulant instead - usually only when the dose is too low.
- **Hops** - 0.5 to 1 g dried herb. For insomnia and calming the nervous system, but is contraindicated in depression.
- **Balm** (melissa) - 2 to 4 g dried herbs for sleep onset insomnia, anxiety, depression and panicky feelings with palpitations.
- **Chamomile** - 1 to 4 g dried herbs calms the nervous system and sedates it.
- **Skullcap** - 1 to 2 g dried herbs sedates the nervous system when tense or hysterical. This herb renews and revives the central nervous system and is useful in exhaustion and depression.

Blends of some can be bought in tablet form from health food stores or a tea can be made of the herb using 30 g (1 oz) to 500 ml of water. This is drunk in divided doses throughout the day.

- **Kava kava** - 70 mg of extract three times daily for nervous anxiety, insomnia, irritability and restlessness, or 210 mg at bedtime for insomnia.
- **Hypericum** - 300 mg of extract three times daily for depression, anxiety and stress. This herb is also effective in nerve pain. Do not combine these last two herbs with drugs which act on the central nervous system.

Essential oils

For massage or adding to the bath.

- **For nervous tension:** bergamot, lavender or neroli and marjoram; or, lavender, ylang ylang, juniper and basil. Both recipes are very relaxing.
- **For anxiety and depression:** bergamot, basil and clary sage.
- **For panic attacks:** clary sage, frankincense, lavender and ylang ylang.

To prepare a bath add a total of 10 to 15 drops of essential oils to half a tub and relax there for 15 to 20 minutes to allow the oils to penetrate the skin.

To prepare a massage oil, add a total of 25 drops to 50 ml (2 oz) of a carrier oil such as avocado or almond. Massage into the back in preference.

You may use any of the following oils at one time - just observe the total dosage.

- **Bergamot** - for tension and depression, as it lightens the mood.
- **Lavender** - for insomnia, depression, headache, palpitation, faintness, aches and pains, fatigue, anxiety, panic, hot flushes, impatience and hypertension.
- **Neroli** - for anxiety, depression, palpitations, nerve spasms and panicky people who get overwrought about nothing.
- **Marjoram** - for insomnia and anxiety, muscle aches and pains.
- **Ylang ylang** - for insomnia and anxiety, depression, tension, frustration, hypertension, tachycardia and all kinds of fears.
- **Juniper** - for stress, anxiety, despondency and the chronic worrier.
- **Basil** - to refresh the mind. It treats depression and nervous exhaustion and is a great nerve tonic.

- **Clary sage** - a wonderful nerve tonic in depression. For nervous, weak and fearful types who are inclined to panic.
- **Geranium** - for feeling unstable, moody and generally stressed. It strengthens the adrenal glands as do basil, rosemary, pine and sage. Geranium also regulates oestrogen.

The olfactory lobe in the brain which interprets smell is connected to our emotional brain (the limbic system). The latter plays a central role in senses such as pain, pleasure, happiness, sadness, joy, fear and sexual feelings as well as in memory and interpreting experience. For this reason, just the smell of some plants or their essential oils can directly affect our emotions. This is why the choice of an oil can also be made according to whether its smell is pleasurable.

Exercise and breathing

Aerobic exercise four times weekly is a very good way of discharging accumulated stress. This can be brisk walking, jogging, swimming, skipping, skating or using a rebounder in the home. Exercise at 60 to 80% of maximum, which means being able to talk whilst exercising and, if you are puffed, then slow down the pace. Tennis and squash are not aerobic as movement is not sustained. One of the reasons people feel so refreshed after aerobic exercise is that adrenalin is released in much greater amounts. Additional benefit is derived from improved circulation, lymph flow and the freeing of tight muscles.

Yoga exercises are good for muscle stretching and learning important breathing techniques which can be used to de-stress the body. Spend a little time each day breathing slowly so that the abdomen is pushed out first followed by the expansion of the lower ribs and finally the upper part of the lungs. Exhale slowly and repeat at a pace which doesn't produce inner tension.

Sunshine through the eyes (without spectacles) daily is important for healthy hormone function and general well-being. In climates with little sunshine, full spectrum lighting in the house is a substitute. Winter depression occurs in many people simply because of the lack of ultraviolet light and using full spectrum lamps has been found to markedly decrease depression, anxiety, hypoactivity, nervousness and other emotional disturbances.

Relaxation

Sleep is vital to health and disturbed sleep patterns need to be rectified as soon as possible. Exercise, a warm bath at bedtimes, flower remedies and the mineral supplements with chamomile tea should help a lot. Everyone, whether stressed or not, should practise a relaxation technique daily. It can be a progressive muscle relaxation, autogenics, abdominal breathing or a biofeedback technique. There are many books on the market which teach these techniques. Try out several methods and follow the one that suits you best.

Most people find the autogenic method very relaxing and Dr. Kay Kermani has published an excellent book on the subject. Very briefly the technique is as follows: Lie down, take a deep breath and then roll your eyes to look at your third eye in the centre of your forehead and then close them. Instruct your arms and legs to go heavy and spend fifteen to twenty seconds on each limb in turn. Focus your entire attention on feeling and mentally seeing the instruction, but do not force it. Do not allow your mind to stray elsewhere and if it does, gently bring it back to what you are saying to yourself. Then continue the instruction to the buttocks, lower back, right up to the shoulders and neck before relaxing the stomach, chest and face. Next instruct all four limbs to become warm and finally cool the forehead which refreshes the mind. The heavy instruction is "my arm is getting heavier and heavier" and the warming instruction is "my arm is getting warmer and warmer". Finally lie still and enjoy the feeling of relaxation while mentally saying "I am completely relaxed and at peace with myself". The whole process takes fifteen to twenty minutes and for those who cannot get off to sleep this works very well. For those who go to sleep easily, relaxation techniques are better done during the daytime.

Everyone to whom I have taught this technique has felt immediate benefit and I have noticed that the rate of breathing and the pulse always become slow and regular. Regular massage to free knotted muscles is very beneficial and, if essential oils are used at the same time, the effect is even greater. Touch is comforting and relaxing in its own right so make the time for a weekly massage.

Meditation

Among the many different types you need to find what suits you best. The Buddhists and raja yoga people teach very good methods free of charge and transcendental meditation (TM) is taught for a fee. Meditation involves concentrating the mind gently on a single thought, word or vision, which stills the chattering thoughts to bring an oasis of peace and calm. It is a chance to listen to your inner self. This should follow on directly from a brief relaxation period and be done three to four times weekly. Even ten minutes a day has a beneficial effect which is cumulative.

Christians who are averse to Eastern meditation techniques can meditate on a saying from the teachings of Jesus such as "I am the way, the truth and the light". This phrase will rapidly take you into a deep meditative state. Meditation is not the same as prayer. Prayer is talking to God while meditation is listening to God. Persevere with the technique because, even if thoughts do crowd the mind, there is benefit from quietude with the intention of meditating and in time it becomes easier.

Aside from relaxation, meditation is used for contacting your higher self so that it can talk to you. After all, when the soul decided to be born into this earthly plane it came with a purpose. Therefore it is really important to spend time away from the clatter of daily life so that the soul can communicate with you, its physical vehicle. Meditation is also time for you to talk to your higher self about your ambitions, fears and wish list. It is time to make affirmations about things you want whether they be to do with self-esteem and confidence or practical assistance in your daily work or home life.

Meditation is the source of all inspiration, confidence, compassion and love. Use this simple tool and discover the enormous benefits.

Changing habits and attitudes

Everyone can change and those who do not accept this will stay in a state of stress until ill health strikes. However, this is the hardest part of all the treatment, as real commitment is necessary to alter stress - inducing habits of a lifetime. Here are a few suggestions:

Take one day at a time and do one thing at a time as far as possible. Make lists of what needs doing, schedule them so that you can cope without feeling stressed and tick them off as you go. This will prevent panic, produce a feeling of control and prevent you from going round in circles without achieving your goals.

Stop making impossible deadlines. Delegate and build in some flexibility to schedules. Always take a full day away from work at the weekend. Do not ignore fatigue or illness as your body is telling you to slow down.

Take regular holidays so that some are occasionally three-day breaks. The long holiday should last no less than two weeks.

Meditate or practise a relaxation technique every day.

Exercise four times weekly.

Eat regularly in relaxed conditions and avoid stimulants and snacks in place of meals.

Spend time each day at a relaxing pastime, be it reading a book not associated with work, watching TV, being social with friends, or doing a creative hobby. Say 'no' to anything which impinges on this area and always ensure adequate sleep at night.

Look at each day in advance with the sole view of finding part of it which generates pleasure in your mind, developing a positive outlook and optimism equating with being happy and relaxed.

Resolve anger and emotional problems through discussion or expression. Do not suppress them as it is important to discuss painful emotions. Work at not over-reacting to small irritations and where these exist, solve the problems instead of reacting to them.

Develop hardiness by first accepting that you alone are responsible for everything in your life and no one else is to blame for situations you do not like. Only then will you be in charge of your life and able to change that which disturbs your equilibrium. Work towards being an optimist, solving your own problems and not being a doormat within the home or workplace.

Recognise the point where duty becomes self-sacrifice and call a halt. Where your expectations conflict with the realities of life, stop and examine ways of living with the reality instead of reacting against it. For instance, if an irritating noise wakes you at 6.00 a.m. every morning, instead of feeling uptight, use ear plugs or get into the habit of taking your daily exercise in the early morning. Alternatively, discuss the problem with the perpetrator. It is acceptable to express your feelings accurately in order to resolve a problem. In this way you control events and do not allow them to damage your health.

Finally, if you like yourself and feel self-confident, your self-esteem will be in good shape and this also increases your hardiness factor. Remember that stress powerfully depresses immune function and that developing hardiness forms a valuable buffer against this and, therefore, against many serious diseases.

So, get a new hairdo, experiment with new ways of dressing, exercise and treat yourself to a weekly massage, facial and manicure. Buy essential oils and use them in the bath and buy an oil burner, as this is all part of feeling beautiful. In menopause, focus on what you want to do for the next few decades, plan the outline and with a feeling of excitement work into it at your own pace. You are a powerful being with a wealth of life experience sitting there waiting to be utilised in the other half of your adult life. Pamper yourself, love yourself, develop confidence in your own abilities and you will gradually look younger because the innate aliveness within you will be given full rein. Believe that you can be whatever you wish and make that belief come true.

Conclusion

We have reached the end of a great deal of information which could be utilised in menopause. It is certainly not necessary to follow everything. However I do suggest that correcting the diet and adding food sources of oestrogen as a matter of routine is very sensible. I would also add vitamin E, a good multivitamin, boron and a low dose calcium/magnesium supplement. Take high dose (1 g) only as a trial to see if it will prove to be the solution to your hot flushes or if your bones need a top up. Use the appropriate flower remedies for emotional distress and treat yourself to a burner, essential oils and a regular massage. I would add a blend of oestrogenic herbs (especially agnus castus if you are suffering flushes) and see if one of the homeopathic remedies matches your personality type or symptoms. If stress is the reason for the flushes then the adrenal glands require the appropriate herbs and vitamins in order to make the hormones come on stream as nature intended. Lifestyle changes are the only way to make theses glands healthy on a long term basis. Get a bone scan to find out if you are at risk for osteoporosis and, if not, don't be panicked by others into unnecessary prevention methods. This book has been written so that you can take charge of your own hormone balance instead of being lead by the nose into a vicious cycle of HRT, disease risk and depleted nutrients, from which you do not know how to break out.

PART 2 - HORMONAL IMBALANCE

1. Premenstrual Syndrome

This condition was first described by a Dr. Robert T. Frank in 1931 and at that time it was called premenstrual tension (PMT).

PMS sufferers endure monthly bouts of a wide variety of symptoms and it is estimated that the incidence is around 40% of all women between puberty and menopause. About 10% have seriously debilitating symptoms. These are cyclical and occur at the same phase of every menstrual cycle. Usually this is immediately premenstrual, but occasionally symptoms begin at ovulation and continue until the start of menses.

The problems vary in individuals, according to the type of PMS, but there is an underlying common hormonal disorder in all, in that oestrogen levels are usually too high and progesterone too low in the post-ovulatory phase. In some, prolactin secretions are elevated and cause breast discomfort, whilst many have raised levels of aldosterone secreted by the adrenal glands. This also contributes to breast tenderness and causes the fluid retention.

PMS has been subdivided into groups, but many women have symptoms of several groups at one time. The four groups are labelled A, C, D and H.

PMS 'A' stands for anxiety. In this, the most common type, the blood oestrogen levels remain high after ovulation and for this reason progesterone synthesis is inhibited. The ovaries work on a feedback system whereby a diminishing blood oestrogen signals the ovaries to increase the progesterone output. Oestrogen is normally broken down by the liver, but if liver function is poor due to excessive carbohydrate and fat in the diet, then oestrogen will continue to circulate and so progesterone secretion remains low. The raised oestrogen affects moods by increasing or inhibiting a variety of chemicals one of which is vitamin B6. The hyperactive feelings arise because oestrogen also causes adrenalin output to increase and the calming brain chemical, dopamine, to be reduced. The knock-on effects of high levels of oestrogen floating around in the blood at inappropriate times is quite amazing.

The results of PMS 'A' are anxiety, weepiness, irritability, anger and hostility, poor concentration and memory, headaches and insomnia. Almost all PMS sufferers fit into this category and the treatment involves inhibiting oestrogen production as well as increasing its removal by the liver from the bloodstream.

An underactive thyroid can also trigger high oestrogen levels. It is the low body temperature in the person with deficient thyroid function that raises the oestrogen. In laboratory studies of 54 women with PMS, 94% were found to have clinical hypo-thyroidism. Thirty four were then given thyroxine with complete relief of symptoms. Since progesterone increases thyroid function, it would seem better to simply alter the oestrogen/progesterone ratio rather than use the heavy duty approach of taking thyroxine.

High oestrogen, aside from causing PMS, is responsible for inhibiting immune function via the thymus gland and for causing constipation, increased fat storage and migraines.

PMS 'C' stands for craving and is caused by low blood sugar levels premenstrually. Again oestrogen is implicated as it competes with the active form of vitamin B6 and lowers glucose tolerance. Low magnesium and deficient synthesis of little tissue hormones called prostaglandin E_1 (PGE_1) from nuts and seeds is involved in PMS 'C'. If the fatty acids in the body are unbalanced by using processed oils, white flour and sugar or, there is a deficiency of vitamins B and C, and the minerals zinc and magnesium, then the body cannot make PGE_1 which is essential for hormonal control. These are the people who need evening primrose or borage oil and magnesium.

The symptoms of PMS 'C' are those of hypoglycaemia; fatigue, tremor, irritability, headaches, dizziness and sugar craving usually occurring around 4.00 p.m. or before breakfast. Weight gain is also a feature. Treatment involves altering the diet and taking magnesium, borage oil, chromium, zinc and vitamin B6.

PMS 'H' stands for hydration meaning fluid retention. Here a magnesium deficiency leads to excessive aldosterone being secreted by the adrenal glands. This hormone causes salt retention and therefore a fluid build up, as well as a further magnesium loss.

It is responsible for the abdominal bloating, breast tenderness and any excessive weight gain. Increased prolactin secretion also plays a part in enlarged painful breasts. Treatment is again aimed at supporting the adrenal and ovarian glands so that they can return to normal function. At the same time, supplements will remove the fluid. This type of PMS is triggered by stress or high serum oestrogen which in turn depletes magnesium. Vitamin B6 will suppress the aldosterone and vitamin E helps with the breast tenderness. Borage and evening primrose oils suppress the prolactin secretion which makes the breasts tender.

PMS 'D' stands for depression and is the least usual. In this case, high stress levels cause high progesterone and low oestrogen. Lead levels have been found to be elevated in many PMS 'D' women and this metal inhibits oestrogen, but not progesterone, and may well be the cause of premenstrual depression. Low magnesium also contributes to lead absorption and retention. Women in this category withdraw from the world, feel confused and forgetful. They are also weepy and unable to sleep at night. Treatment is dependent on the cause, but is also aimed at supporting the adrenal glands and altering the response to stress.

Treatment

Vitamin B6 in higher levels after ovulation will reduce the oestrogen and prolactin as well as increasing progesterone. It suppresses the adrenal secretion of aldosterone and so beneficially affects water retention. B6 is necessary for all problems relating to metabolism, hormonal production and red and white blood cells. It is vital for controlled function of the nervous system and muscles as well as the sodium/potassium balance and normal behavioural patterns. A general B deficiency leads to diminished liver function and therefore its reduced ability to clear oestrogen adequately. Most studies indicate that 80% of women experience an overall improvement in PMS symptoms with 80 to 200 mg of vitamin B6 daily. If the dosage is lower than 50 mg, the results tend to be poor. Vitamin B6 will also prevent premenstrual acne from flaring up.

Magnesium works hand in glove with B6 in so many vital functions that the two should always be given together. Studies have indicated that the only situations of toxicity from high levels of B6 arose when magnesium was not also given, and neurological toxicity only occurs if B6 is in the range of 2,000 mg daily (short term) or 500 mg daily (long term). A study of patients prone to kidney stones who were given 500 mg of B6 daily for three years from 1981 to 1984 indicated no side effects, as these people were also taking magnesium. In a study at a London hospital where 630 patients were given 80 to 200 mg of B6 daily no side effects were noted and PMS symptoms improved by 70 to 80%. On the other hand, magnesium, given alone in controlled studies, has reduced mood swings by 80%, and breast symptoms and weight gain by nearly 100%. The two together have remarkable effects in most women. Magnesium deficiency causes a decrease in vitamin B6 activity.

In a study reported in France with 196 women, magnesium supplements improved nervous tension by 89%, painful breasts by 96%, fluid retention by 95% and headaches by 43%. The magnesium dose was very high and given for only one week prior to menstruation. Magnesium is low in the red blood cells of PMS women - serum levels do not accurately indicate magnesium status in anyone.

A magnesium deficiency can contribute to oestrogen excess as this mineral is necessary for the metabolism of oestrogen in the liver. Magnesium is also essential in adequate amounts so that progesterone and oestrogen can bind to tissue receptors and therefore have an active effect in the body. This mineral is necessary for B vitamins to convert to their active form and omega 6 oils to convert to GLA. It is also essential for controlling the amount of sodium and fluid retained in the body by the adrenal glands, that is, magnesium prevents any excess.

Manganese - In a study reported in 1993, this mineral was given with calcium to ten women with menstrual problems. The result was a marked improvement in moods, behaviour, fluid retention and painful periods. Manganese appeared to be particularly important in regulating moods and pain. This mineral also works hand in hand with zinc.

Evening primrose and **borage oils** contains GLA which is eventually converted to prostaglandin E_1, the little tissue hormones which play a major part in maintaining hormonal balances. It is particularly useful for the breast symptoms but needs to be taken for several months before improvement is obvious. Controlled studies also conclude that these oils will improve all PMS symptoms by a significant percentage. One group of women with severe PMS who had failed to respond to vitamin B6, started taking evening primrose oil at a high dose just a few days before symptoms were due: 61% experienced total relief and 23% only partial. Cases of severe fluid retention failed to respond.

Vitamin E at the rate of 200 IU. daily increases progesterone levels and improves mood changes and the mastalgia by its regulatory effect on hormones. One study found that 300 IU daily had significant benefit in PMS 'A' and 600 IU for PMS 'C' and 'D'. Only fluid retention was not altered. Vitamin E inhibits the inflammatory prostaglandin E_2 produced from eating meat and increases the anti-inflammatory prostaglandin E_1. A mixture of vitamin E and B6, zinc and GLA will ensure mastalgia symptoms disappear, as long as the diet is also improved.

Oestrogen clearance is inhibited by high levels of simple carbohydrate like sugar, white flour, processed cereals and everything made from them. Statistics indicate that PMS sufferers on average eat at least three times more sugar, refined carbohydrate and dairy products than other women. Because of this they also have very low levels of many essential nutrients. For instance a deficiency of vitamin B2 causes an excessive accumulation of oestrogen in the blood - the liver requires this vitamin for hormone clearance. The minerals which are usually deficient in PMS women are magnesium, zinc and manganese. Low levels of magnesium are explained by the fact that women with PMS 'A' consume five times more dairy products than non-sufferers and the high calcium inhibits magnesium absorption. Sugar increases magnesium loss through the kidneys and this interferes with the liver's ability to deactivate oestrogen. Simply changing the diet to high levels of wholefoods containing vegetable protein will alone increase oestrogen clearance through the liver. Vegetarians clear two to three times more oestrogen than meat eaters, and it should be remembered that farmed meat contains high levels of synthetic oestrogen which exacerbates PMS symptoms. The presence of healthy micro-flora like lactobacillus in the intestines increases the breakdown of oestrogen in the liver. However, the presence of animal fat stimulates the growth of unhealthy micro-flora that have the ability to transform oestrogen back to its original active form.

Anything which improves liver function will help reduce PMS symptoms. The sulphur amino acid, methionine, is very effective here, as is dandelion herb. The flavonoid quercetin inhibits oestrogen synthesis by competing with it in biochemical reactions.

Diet

- **Protein** from vegetable sources, i.e., dried peas, beans, lentils, soya beans, whole grains, nuts and seeds and especially oats, millet, barley and buckwheat.
- A little **oily fish** as a source of protein and the essential polyunsaturated oil, omega 3. Vegetarians should use flaxseed (linseed) oil for their omega 3.
- **Seeds** of all kinds, and walnuts for the essential polyunsaturated oils, omega 6 and 3. Seeds are always better sprouted, but in very hot climates that is not possible.
- Plenty of **raw fruit** and vegetables (especially green leafy ones), garlic, watercress, artichokes and pineapple. Fruit or vegetables should make up 75% of your plate at every meal. This can be reduced proportionally if millet, soya beans or buckwheat form a significant part of the diet. These are all alkaline forming foods. Do remember to include a variety of root vegetables routinely.
- **Potassium** rich foods: potatoes, spinach and other greens, parsnip, pumpkin and tomatoes, pulses, avocadoes, bananas, nectarines and mangoes.

- **Chromium** rich foods for blood sugar control: Brewer's yeast, egg yolk, oatmeal, wheat germ, whole grains, mushrooms, lettuce, tomatoes, beans, onions, liver, clams and cheese.
- **Chromium** rich **herbs** - caraway, coriander, mace, cinnamon, nutmeg, poppy seeds, cumin, cloves and bayleaves.
- **Iron** rich foods: nuts, seeds, whole grains and small amounts of molasses in cooking. Also free-range eggs, apricots, peaches, bananas and raisins. Remember that dried fruits are concentrated carbohydrate sources so should be eaten in very small amounts. Vegetables are high in iron but we absorb very little of it. Vitamin C increases iron absorption from greens.
- **Seaweed** for iodine, calcium, magnesium and other minerals.
- A daily **vegetable juice** which, in addition to the usual carrots, has beetroot and dark greens for liver detoxification. This is part of the 75% alkaline forming foods.

The diet should be low in fat, protein, simple carbohydrate, sugar and salt, but high in complex carbohydrate (whole grains, pulses, vegetables and fruit). Eat only unprocessed food and take a complex carbohydrate snack such as almonds or yoghurt with fruit between meals to maintain steady blood sugar levels once you are in the premenstrual phase of your cycle. Do not reach for chocolate or processed food snacks between meals because these will raise your blood sugar temporarily - you will plummet down into low blood sugar fairly soon after. A breakfast of oatmeal porridge and a little low-fat cow's milk or nut milk will feed sugar into the blood at a slow controlled rate all morning. Eat either whole grains or pulses at every meal, for instance, brown rice, wholegrain pasta, dark rye bread, dried peas or beans or tofu. This releases glucose into the bloodstream in steady amounts, instead of the rush you get with chocolate or sugar.

Avoid

Smoking, as nicotine aggravates menstrual disorders.

Sugar, white flour, white rice, processed cereals and everything made from them.

Added salt as it increases magnesium loss and fluid retention.

Coffee for five days prior to menstruation.

Soft drinks and all processed foods.

All margarines and oils not genuinely cold pressed. Use extra virgin olive oil for dressings and salads.

All farmed meat and fowl initially, unless free of added hormones. In any case, animal protein increases the amount of oestrogen absorbed, as meat eaters have intestinal bacteria which make their own variety of this hormone. This is then absorbed unless the fibre content of the diet is very high.

Reduce

Coffee, tea and alcohol.

Honey, dried fruit, molasses and fruit juice, as they are very concentrated forms of carbohydrate.

Milk and other dairy products, as they interfere with magnesium absorption.

Total fat intake and all animal protein.

Supplements of value

For all types of PMS:

- **Vitamin B6** - 100 mg daily and increase to twice daily immediately premenstrually if necessary.
- **B complex** - 25 mg daily. A multivitamin/mineral supplement with this low-dose B complex also supplies trace minerals like selenium which are important to good health and important as co-factors to the specific supplements suggested for PMS.
- **Magnesium** - 400 to 800 mg daily, as citrate or aspartate or amino acid chelate.
- **Calcium** - 1000 mg daily in the same form as the magnesium. Take this at night.

- **Vitamin C** - 500 mg daily.
- **Beta carotene** - 15 mg daily in the second half of the menstrual cycle may improve PMS headaches and fluid retention.
- **Zinc** - 15 mg daily as citrate or amino acid chelate.
- **Manganese** - 5 to 10 mg daily.
- **Vitamin E** - 200 IU daily.

Many quality manufacturers make supplements especially designed for PMS, which contain all of the above and sometimes other minerals and herbs as well.

PMS 'A'

- **Quercetin** - 400 mg twice daily to inhibit oestrogen.
- **Methionine** - 1 g twice daily to increase oestrogen clearance by the liver if necessary.

PMS 'C'

- **Evening primrose** - 500 mg three times daily or half dose **borage oil.**
- **GTF chromium or chromium polynicotinate** - 200 mcg daily for sugar control.
- **Methionine** - as above.

PMS 'H'

- **Evening primrose** - 500 mg three times daily or half dose **borage oil.**
- **Licorice root** - 1 g three times daily premenstrually only.

PMS 'D'

- **Avoid vitamin B6** in the week before menses.
- **Check for lead levels** by hair testing and follow a heavy metal chelation programme if necessary.
- **High carbohydrate** and **low protein** at the evening meal will improve depression.

It is my experience with patients, that PMS can be totally eradicated by changing the diet and taking the indicated supplements and herbs. Eventually the added nutrients are no longer needed as the corrected diet will maintain a symptom free menstrual cycle.

Herbs

Agnus castus - A mediterranean herb which regulates hormones by its effect on the pituitary gland. It reduces the follicle stimulating hormone and increases the luteinizing hormone so that the hormone balance swings towards producing more progesterone. Agnus castus can be bought in tablets from health food stores. Take 0.5 to 4 g daily or make an infusion with one teaspoon of ripe berries in one cup of water three times daily. This is fairly bitter - the tincture is more palatable at the rate of one teaspoon twice daily between meals.

Bupleurum sedative pills - is a Chinese formula containing bupleurum, paeonia, dong quai, poria, atractylodes, ginger, licorice and peppermint. Studies indicate that six out of ten women taking this commercial product experience a marked improvement in mood swings, cramps, breast pain and fluid retention. This formula also regulates periods. It can be bought in Chinese herbal stores as tablets.

Oestrogen herbs will bind to receptors and so reduce oestrogen function in the body. Choose one listed under "Phytotherapy" and make an infusion to drink daily.

Homeopathy

Dosage of remedies is 30C one to three times daily on PMS days for up to seven days. Do not repeat a dosage while symptoms are in abeyance. The closer the symptoms match, the more effective the remedy. Choosing the wrong one will neither harm nor improve.

Folliculinum - 30c monthly or daily if necessary immediately premenstrually for breast pain, fluid retention, weight gain and mood swings. The person may have had a repressed or very disciplined childhood. This remedy is made from synthetic oestrogen and will remove symptoms of excess oestrogen.

Sepia - This personality type is irritable and easily offended, weepy, sad and anxious. She craves sweets or salt. Symptoms include irregular periods which may be late and light or early and heavy, accompanied by a pain of a bearing down nature. There may be a painful vagina and possibly pains shooting upwards. She may be averse to sex and to loved ones. Feels better with strenuous exercise.

Lachesis - For painful breasts and fluid retention. Periods are short and light. Symptoms are worse first thing in the morning. The left ovary may be painful and swollen. Low back pain. Needs sex as an outlet for emotions. This person is very talkative and can't bear tight clothes.

Pulsatilla - is prone to floods of tears and needs sympathy. Painful breasts, and irregular delayed periods. Pain feels like a downward pressure. Tired feeling, chilliness and nausea. Nervous debility will cause a late or missed period.

Lycopodium - is typically depressed, lacking self-confidence and bad tempered. Fear of breaking down under stress. Constipated and flatulent and craves sweet food. Overeats and bloats. Menses late, long and profuse. Right ovary may be painful.

Nux vomica - the irritable, malicious or quarrelsome individual who craves sweet, fat and rich food. Gains weight easily and has irregular periods with pain in the sacrum.

Nat. mur. - for fluid retention and breast swelling. This woman also suffers heavy painful periods or missed periods. Irritable, sad and wants to be alone to cry. Worse for sympathy. Gets in a state about trifles. Menstrual headaches. Craves salt, is very thirsty and dislikes fats and slimy things like oysters. This woman is very sensitive and will avoid emotional pain at all costs. Because she cannot tolerate rejection, ridicule or humiliation she builds a wall of invulnerability around her. This wall also helps to prevent her from absorbing the pain of others. She is mentally strong but emotionally introverted. If the emotional control breaks down she becomes irrational.

Cimicifuga - Pain immediately before menses which may shoot up and down the front of the thighs or across the pelvis from hip to hip. Heavy periods and there may be afterpains.

Calc. Carb. - painful swollen breasts, heavy periods with cutting pains in the uterus. Sweating, headache. chilliness and dizziness. Increased sexual desire. Burning and itching of parts before and after menstruation.

Mag. phos. - spasms of pain, which feel better for bending double, pressure and a hot water bag.

Borax - Nausea and the pain radiates down the thigh.

Graphites - Periods late and are accompanied by constipation. They may be light with itching beforehand. Sweats and morning nausea during menstruation. Swollen, tender breasts.

Kali carb. - Very tense and exhausted. Symptoms worse from 2.00 to 4.00 a.m. Pains go from the lower back down through the buttocks with cutting pains in the abdomen. Much bloating of the abdomen with fluid. Spotting after the period. Difficult first menses in young girls.

Chamomilla - severe cramping pains and anger about unfair situations.

Flower essences

Refer to chapter Part 1 - chapter 19 on stress, as there are many flower remedies which will help in PMS.

Essential oils

The chapter on stress lists a very broad range of oils which will bring relief from PMS. The ones which especially relate to hormone balance are geranium, rosemary, basil, cypress, fennel, eucalyptus and clary sage.

2. Dysmenorrhoea

Painful menstruation is common to many women, but for some it can be very severe indeed. Discomfort for one or two days is normal and can be treated with a homeopathic, herbal or mineral remedy. For some women, a hot water bag will soothe the cramps. However when period pain persists, varying from a dull ache in the back to severe cramping pains in the abdomen, the situation may be completely debilitating for hours. To add to their misery, some women experience nausea and vomiting, fainting and dizziness. Anxiety makes the whole situation worse.

Sometimes, dysmenorrhoea is due to hormone imbalance which is covered in the chapter on PMS. However, more often a simple remedy will solve the problem. You just need to find the one which suits you.

Exercise is important because cramps are due to increased production of the inflammatory prostaglandins (PGF_2 alpha and PGE_2) in the uterine tissue. Both can be reduced quite dramatically with vigorous exercise. However the exercise does need to be quite strenuous and on a daily basis. Walking in the hills is as effective as a workout in the gym. PGF_2 and PGE_2 are formed from arachidonic acid (often the result of too much animal protein being eaten or over-exposure to processed polyunsaturates) and are released to create mayhem when the endometrium is shed as the monthly bleed. (You will notice that a theme recurring throughout this book, is the damage done by animal protein and fat in most types of hormone imbalance).

Excessive PGF_2 and PGE_2 also occurs when the anti-inflammatory PGE_1 and PGE_3 are not around to exert control over them. These little tissue hormones are made from the EPA in oil from fish like salmon, mackerel and sardines and the GLA in evening primrose or borage oil. The precursor oils of these active chemicals are found in flaxseeds, soya beans and walnuts, sunflower, pumpkin and sesame seeds, but these can be prevented from exerting any activity in the body by stress, processed grains, sugar products and by the usual range of processed fats and oils found in the supermarkets. The packaged products covering rows of shelves in these shops contain considerable amounts of all these so-called foods. Is it any wonder that hormone imbalance is increasingly becoming a major problem for such a vast number of women? Avoiding processed foods requires a major shift for many people. If you are one of these, do not despair - work into it and you will find it really not so difficult to go back to a natural way of eating. In time, you will find that you actually prefer it and feel somewhat below par when you deviate from it for any length of time.

Another factor concerning polyunsaturated oils is that the ratio between the omega 3 and 6 types consumed in our diets is also important. Because of all the processed polyunsaturates used in foods, dressings and cooking oils we tend to ingest far too much omega 6 - even these very harmful processed types count in the ratio! In comparison, we do not eat enough omega 3 oils in the form of flaxseed oil and EPA in oily fish. A Danish study in 1995 involving 220 women suffering from painful menses, determined that not only did high levels of EPA from fish oils significantly reduce pain but the ratio between the intake omega 3 and 6 intake was even more important for a successful outcome. So, if you want to prevent your uterine cramps, stop using those poisonous processed polyunsaturated oils and dressings from the supermarket. Get your omega 6 oils from walnuts and seeds, cook with extra virgin oil or coconut oil and eat more oily fish like sardines, mackerel, salmon and herrings. Coconut oil neither raises nor lowers cholesterol - it is a neutral innocent bystander. This is scientific fact. Sadly people prefer to believe the false advertising of those who produce and sell the petrochemically processed polyunsaturated oils which are poisoning humanity.

Treatment

Diet

If you suffer from dysmenorrhoea it is wise to shift to a largely vegetarian diet with just a little fish until your symptoms are corrected on a long-term basis. The PMS diet (see p. 104) is a good basic one to follow, but if you do not suffer with low blood sugar premenstrually, it is not necessary to eat between meals. Take particular care to reduce the foods which increase inflammatory prostaglandins (animal protein) and be sure to include those that increase the helpful ones - unroasted and unsalted seeds and walnuts, soya products and oily fish, if you are not totally vegetarian. Protein and fat must be reduced while complex carbohydrate from pulses and whole grains need to be increased.

Supplements of value

- **GLA** as **evening primrose oil** - 1500 mg daily or as **borage oil** at half this dosage.
- **Flaxseed oil** - 3,000 mg daily or you may need high dose MaxEPA from fish oil - 3 to 6 g daily.
- **Vitamin B3** - 100 mg twice daily as niacinamide for a few days premenstrually and during the pain of menses may be worth trying. Take vitamin C and bioflavonoids with it.
- **Vitamin B6** - 100 to 200 mg daily for one week premenstrually and 50 mg daily for the rest of the month.
- **Magnesium** - 200 mg twice daily.
- **Mag. phos. and calc. phos.** - tissue salts, taken hourly if necessary will often eradicate cramps when they occur.
- **Vitamin C** - 500 mg 3 times daily with bioflavonoids.
- **Vitamin E** - 200 IU daily.
- **Iron** - 15 mg daily if the cramps are due to iron deficient anaemia. Get a blood test to find out.
- **Evening primrose or borage oil** produces PGE_1 to balance hormones and block inflammatory prostaglandins, while flaxseed oil or EPA provides PGE_3. Some women find that they form PGE_3 better from fish oil and take MaxEPA in high doses until the diet is corrected and the body is blocking the inflammatory chemicals.

- **Vitamin B6 and magnesium** are important for everyone to take all month, but the dose can be increased in the week before menstruation and until the cramps cease. In time these two nutrients will assist in balancing your hormones so that cramps cease to be a problem. Then, low maintenance doses will be appropriate. I always give zinc to my patients as well because all menstrual disorders will benefit from it.

Magnesium is a muscle relaxant and a vasodilator and many studies have been published demonstrating the efficacy of this mineral against uterine cramps. Magnesium also has the ability to reduce levels of PGF_2 in the blood which is high in women with dysmenorrhoea.

Vitamin B6 balances hormones, reduces fluid retention and increases the movement of magnesium into the uterine muscle where it has its relaxing effect. Guy Abraham, who was responsible for categorising PMS into the four types, has done many controlled trials using various nutrients in hormonal disorders. In 1978 he reported that a group of women with low red blood cell magnesium were given 100 mg of magnesium with vitamin B6 four times daily all month and at two hourly intervals for pain during menses. In four to six months these women experienced a gradual reduction in menstrual pain until they became normal. Studies using vitamin B3 have also proved beneficial, but this is probably only because of this vitamin's ability to dilate blood vessels and so improve the flow of nutrients to the uterine muscle.

- **Bioflavonoids** are often helpful along with higher dose Vitamin C and they certainly have the effect of reducing heavy bleeding. Rutin is the one to look for. This bioflavonoid acts by strengthening blood vessel walls and their elasticity. However it is an effective contraceptive in high dose so do not take it if you are trying to become pregnant.

- **Vitamin E** has been found to reduce cramps in controlled studies. Nearly 70% of a test group of women experienced relief within two months of taking about 150 IU daily for just ten days premenstrually. This vitamin also has the ability to balance hormones.

Herbs

- **Black haw** and **cramp bark -** are two herbs that have anti-spasmodic effects and are known as uterine sedatives. These tend to be used for pain relief.
- **False unicorn, squaw vine, black cohosh, and life root** - are uterine tonics which increase the ability of the uterus to shed the endometrium ready for a clean start in the following cycle. These herbs are used all month as a tonic.
- **Wild yam** - is anti-spasmodic and for ovarian pain.
- **Pasque flower** - relaxes nervous tension and spasm and combines well with cramp bark.
- **White dead nettle** - improves uterine circulation and will stop spasm. This herb needs to be taken at the rate of one teaspoon daily (in divided doses) for several months to eradicate the problem.

Two good recipes to use for pain relief are:

A. 2 parts cramp bark and 1 part black cohosh and 1 part pasque flower, and B. equal parts of squaw vine, wild yam, cramp bark or black haw.

Mix these either as tinctures and take one teaspoon four times daily if necessary, or use dried herbs and make an infusion with 30 g (1 oz) to 500 ml of water and drink as three cups throughout the day. Alternatively, as this tea does not taste too good, you may prefer to choose tablets from one of the many proprietary blends available in good health food shops.

Others

Use a hot water bag on the abdomen or make a hot fomentation by frying two cups of salt, placing this between heated cloth and putting it on the abdomen with the hot water bag on top. Do not burn your skin by making this too hot.

Use an infrared lamp for fifteen minutes before massaging the abdomen with essential oils in a carrier oil. This helps any clots to pass. Do not put the oil on before using the lamp.

Drink ginger and chamomile tea while you are resting in bed with your heat treatment. Hot chamomile tea brings rapid relief from spasm when sipped slowly, and ginger relieves nausea and colic as well as stimulating the circulation to the reproductive organs.

Acupuncture, chiropractic and osteopathic treatment are very helpful for relieving pain.

Essential oils

See chapter Part 1 - chapter 8 in the menopause section to understand how to mix and use essential oils.

- **Chamomile** and **parsley** go well together for the antispasmodic and calming effect; they also help to release any clots and improve the menstrual flow.
- **Clary sage** - is a female tonic oil which is useful in painful periods and all kinds of menstrual disorders.
- **Cypress** - is a powerful anti-spasmodic and has a great affinity for the female reproductive system. It also has an astringent effect and so is useful in heavy periods.
- **Jasmine** and **marjoram** - are antispasmodic and also have a great affinity for the nervous system in terms of relieving anxiety and depression.
- **Peppermint** - is cooling and antispasmodic, relieves nausea and has a calming effect on the nervous system.

Homeopathy

Dose 6C or 30C hourly, if necessary, for up to ten doses:

- **Chamomilla -** for severe cramping pains with clots, particularly if irritable and restless.
- **Gelsemium** - For spasms of sharp pain in the abdomen and especially the lower back; and the type of cramps which fit gelsemium also feel better following the application of a hot compress.
- **Mag. phos.** - works in cramps that are better for heat application and bending double.

- **Viburnum** - For late, light periods with a sudden onset pain that spreads all over the abdomen and extends into the thighs.
- **Pulsatilla** - For scanty or profuse flow, with nausea and vomiting accompanying cutting and tearing pain. Pulsatilla is inclined to weepiness and in need of comforting.
- **Nux vomica** - For long periods with excessive irritability, exhaustion and constipation.
- **Cimicifuga** - The cramps feel like labour pains and the period is preceded by headaches.

3. Menorrhagia And Fibroids

Menorrhagia, the medical term for excessively heavy periods, has several possible causes. There may be too much oestrogen in the body in relationship to progesterone or there may be uterine fibroids, ovarian cysts, endometriosis or serious disease. It is important to find the cause before deciding to follow only natural therapies. Hypothyroidism, which means a sluggish thyroid, is a possible reason for the oestrogen not being cleared from the blood so that progesterone can come on stream at the correct time. The presence of too much oestrogen means that the endometrium is overly built up, with the result that there is a lot to be removed in the menses.

Fibroids are a major cause of heavy periods, but they can be destroyed by herbs. Opting for a hysterectomy instead is a sad decision, as fibroids are rarely cancerous. However, they do seem to be oestrogen dependent for growth and treatment involves reducing this hormone with herbs. Butterbur is a herb which shrinks fibroids and tumours of all kinds - even from grapefruit size. A very large one will require treatment for about a year. Dong quai is a herb which should be avoided where fibroids exist, as it may stimulate their growth.

The long-term effects of a hysterectomy include accelerated ageing of the ovaries, depression and negative effects on pheromone secretions, arousal, orgasm and libido. Any woman who undergoes this surgery will also enter menopause about five years earlier than average. Statistics published in the last year, show that if a 35-year-old woman has a hysterectomy, she has a sevenfold increased risk of heart attack than a woman who keeps her uterus. Many of my patients choosing natural treatments instead of a hysterectomy, have had before and after scans which clearly indicate the effectiveness of herbs, supplements and a healthy diet. Dramatic shrinkage has been shown to occur within three months. Agnus castus herb changes the balance of hormones towards a progesterone emphasis so this will also help to shrink fibroids.

Dietary reasons for heavy periods include an imbalance of those prostaglandins discussed in other chapters, whereby PGF_2 is in control and this causes heavy bleeding and pain. Certain nutritional deficiencies can result in fragile capillaries, which is sometimes the sole reason for heavy bleeds. IUDs (intrauterine devices) can also be responsible for pain and heavy menses. Whatever the cause, the fact remains that it is a wretched nuisance every month, especially as some women dare not leave the house on the first few days of the period. I hope some of these ideas will relieve this situation for you.

Treatment

Diet

Follow the recommendations for dysmenorrhoea.

Supplements of value

- **Vitamin C** - 500 mg three times daily.
- **Bioflavonoids** - 250 mg three times daily.
- **Vitamin A** - 50,000 to 100,000 IU for two weeks prior to the period. Studies indicate that many women with heavy periods have considerably lower levels of vitamin A than those with normal menstruation.
- **Chlorophyll** - 25 mg for vitamin K.
- **GLA** as **evening primrose oil** - 2000 mg daily or half dose **borage oil.**

Giving the vitamin C, bioflavonoids and vitamin A together has been shown in a study to improve heavy bleeding in some women by 100% while others improved by at least 50%.

- **Iron** - 10 to 20 mg depending on whether you are low in haemoglobin. It is important to check serum ferritin levels with a blood test, as one study of women with heavy periods found that, although haemoglobin was normal, serum ferritin was significantly below normal. In other words these women were iron deficient in spite of having normal haemoglobin. Several studies have indicated successful eradication of heavy bleeding after a period of iron supplementation. It would seem that the iron deficiency caused by the excessive blood loss in turn caused further heavy bleeding.

If you have heavy periods or fibroids, you may also have a hormone imbalance, so other nutrients like vitamin B6, magnesium, vitamin E or zinc may be necessary. You can also choose to balance your hormones with herbs or homeopathy. This subject is covered in PMS.

Herbs

- **Shepherd's purse** - is used in uterine haemorrhage to stop the bleeding. It is a uterine stimulant which at the same time has an astringent effect on the blood flow. Infuse 1 to 2 teaspoons in a cup for 15 minutes three times daily.
- **Beth root, greater periwinkle and American cranesbill** are all good astringents and these three may be combined successfully. Add 1 to 2 teaspoons of one herb or a mix of these herbs and boil a few minutes only before drinking three times daily.
- **Squaw vine or life root** - as an infusion for toning the uterus.
- **White dead nettle** - is astringent to the uterus, improves the circulation there and has a tonic effect on the reproductive organs.
- **Agnus castus (chaste tree)** - Take 0.5 to 4 g daily for balancing the hormones or crush one to two teaspoons of the ripe berries and use them for an infusion three times daily. This is important if you have fibroids as it will encourage the progesterone phase of the cycle rather than the oestrogen one.
- **Butterbur** - For uterine fibroids take 40 to 80 mg of the extract or 1 to 2 ml of tincture three times daily. The tincture is widely available as "Petasites" by Bioforce.

Essential oils

- **Cypress -** has astringent and styptic properties and has great affinity for the female reproductive system.
- **Geranium -** is an astringent oil, relieves pain and uplifts and soothes the nervous system. This oil also balances hormones.

Homeopathy

Dose with 30C 6 to 8 hourly if necessary during menses.

- **China -** for clotting which is dark in colour, abdominal distension, headache, dizziness and paleness in the face.
- **Sabina -** for heavy periods with pain like those experienced in labour. Emotional upsets increase the bleeding and these women are usually overweight. The blood loss is heavy and bright red. Uterine pains extend down the thighs. This is a good remedy for a threatened miscarriage.
- **Ipecac. -** for when there is bright red blood loss with nausea. Pain is felt from navel to uterus.
- **Belladonna -** for bright red blood, dragging pains, throbbing headache and the face is hot and red.
- **Calcarea -** for use when there are cutting pains in the lower back and abdomen, copious menses, pallor and chill, as well as itching of parts before and after menstruation. Breast tenderness.
- **Ferrum phos. -** for dark, watery flooding. Face pale but it flushes easily on exertion.
- **Kali carb. -** for a heavy, thin watery bleed with exhaustion and cold extremities.
- **Borax -** for early, profuse and painful periods. The bleeding is heaviest at night.
- **Lachesis -** is especially useful for severe cramping pains, clots and irritability which improve once the flow gets going. Hot fluhes may also feature.

- **Sepia** - for heavy loss with bearing down pain as though everything would fall out. Bursts of irritability.
- **Pulsatilla** - for intermittent flooding which is associated with pain in the lower back and abdomen. Person is weepy and the symptoms are changeable.

4. Endometriosis

This is a condition born out of general toxicity, but it is also associated with low immunity, candida albicans, the tendency to infections, stress and hormone imbalance. Stress will cause hormonal imbalance and immune dysfunction and these conditions provide an environment in which endometriosis thrives. Fragments of the endometrium (lining of the uterus) spread into the vagina, fallopian tubes and finally into the pelvic cavity outside the reproductive system. Once there, these particles are sensitive to stimulation by the female hormones and so they grow and thicken every month as though inside the uterus. The problem is exacerbated by the fact that when it is time for the endometrium to be shed as a menstrual flow, the faulty overgrowth has nowhere to go if it is in the pelvic cavity. This results in irritation and eventual scarring of the surrounding tissue.

The symptoms are *pain* which worsens towards the end of the period, heavy periods and even painful intercourse. In time the pain may become constant and very severe. Women are sometimes given a course of a testosterone-type drug in an attempt to stop the build up of endometrium by oestrogen so that the body can get to grips with absorbing the displaced tissue. Pregnancy often solves the problem by stopping the monthly cycles of oestrogen; endometriosis is oestrogen dependent.

Other symptoms may be fatigue, depression and diarrhoea, constipation or other intestinal disturbances. In some cases, there is a complete lack of pain and so the condition develops silently.

Doctors commonly prescribe a D & C and, in severe cases, a complete hysterectomy will be advised if there is much scarring of the tubes. Where infection develops, a constant battle with antibiotics ensues. This destroys the healthy bacteria in the reproductive tract and other problems like candida albicans may develop. In fact endometriosis is frequently associated with candida, which must be treated before a healthy reproductive tract can become a reality.

In natural medicine we use herbs very successfully. However it is absolutely vital to do a very thorough detoxification of the whole body by means of a juice fast. This is followed by an extended period of eating mainly fruits and vegetables with brown rice, millet, quinoa or oats for those who are very hungry.

Treatment

Diet

Follow an anti-candida diet if this fungus is present. If stress is a contributing factor in causing or maintaining the endometriosis then read Part 1, chapter 19 and incorporate the guidelines which resonate with you. Otherwise start with a juice fast for five days, followed by two weeks of only fruit and vegetables as salads, soups or in a lightly steamed form. "You don't have to feel unwell" has detailed information in these areas.

Basically a juice fast involves drinking freshly squeezed fruits or vegetables and drinking a large glass every two to three hours. Mineral water is important and herbal tea is also permitted. Canned and packaged juices are strictly forbidden. The juices should include beetroot (red beet) and some dark greens for a liver detoxification. Lemon juice also detoxifies the liver. In cold climates, vegetable broth is a good idea twice a day, but no fibre should be present. The soup needs to be simmered very slowly so all the nutrients are released from the fibre which is then thrown away. Following five days of this, add whole fruit for breakfast on day 6, a salad for lunch on day 7 and cooked vegetables for dinner on day 8. Continue in this manner with as many juices as you wish as well until you have done a twenty day detoxification.

The next stage is to add one food group each day until you are back on a healthy, wholefood diet rich in fruit, vegetables, wholegrains, pulses, nuts and seeds (unroasted and unsalted), with small amounts of fish, egg and occasional meat if you must. Stay with drinking fruit and vegetable juices, herbal tea and mineral water instead of perhaps renewing a love of coffee and tea. Try miso for a change and take unhealthy drinks sparingly.

Avoid

Boron supplements as these increase oestrogen.

All dairy products

All farmed meat unless guaranteed organic and free of hormones.

All processed food - everything fresh and natural. Avoid sugar.

All pesticides as they have oestrogenic activity.

Reduce citrus fruits and wheat as they contain substances which may mimic oestrogen.

Supplements of value

The supplements suggested in Part 2, chapter 1 on PMS which balance hormones are all very important in endometriosis. Make sure the vitamin E is 800 IU daily and increase the vitamin C to 6,000 to 10,000 mg daily in divided doses. If this amount of' vitamin C causes any nervous irritation take it in the form of calcium ascorbate. The calcium component will prevent the acidity of vitamin C from irritating. In any case, this amount is unlikely to create problems. Include GLA, magnesium, zinc, vitamin B6 and B complex, as in PMS. Vitamin B2 is vital for clearing oestrogen through the liver and it is also an essential component in adrenal gland function and therefore in stress. Vitamin B6 is needed for progesterone production and zinc is vital for immune function. In fact the whole B complex is necessary before the liver can break down oestrogen. Double-blind research projects involving women with endometriosis have consistently indicated that the above nutrients lead to a significant improvement in symptoms.

It has also been demonstrated that EPA supplements significantly reduce the growth of endometriosis by combating the pain-inducing inflammatory chemicals, PGE_2 and PGF_2 alpha. Kelp tablets or seaweed are important. If the liver is sluggish, it is wise to take some methionine to help it clear oestrogen correctly.

Many manufacturers make up blends of vitamins and minerals specific to menstrual problems, so it is possible to avoid taking a fistful of tablets at every meal. A multivitamin/mineral supplement provides co-factors which act with the above mentioned nutrients and this is very important if you are taking single supplements for any length of time.

Herbs

A good blend is as follows:

- **Echinacea** - stimulates immunity and is effective against infections and fungus.
- **Golden seal** - is also effective against fungus and bacteria. It has a healing effect on mucous membranes, is anti-inflammatory and has a mild laxative effect. This must be avoided if pregnancy is suspected as it stimulates the uterine muscle. These two herbs deal with any infection or fungus.
- **Squaw vine** - is an astringent tonic to the uterus and plays a part in balancing hormones.
- **Blessed thistle** - is astringent and antibacterial.
- **False unicorn** - is a uterine tonic and hormone balancer.
- **Wild yam** -is antispasmodic and therefore helps to relieve pain.
- **Parsley** - stimulates release of excess endometrium and is a mild diuretic.

Mix all these tinctures together and take 1 teaspoon three times daily. You can also buy the herbs in dried form, powder them in your blender and put this into empty capsules or into some food which will hide the taste! Medicinal herbs seldom taste pleasant. Agnus castus and dong quai are other useful herbs. I suggest you do take agnus castus along with the above blend as it will reduce the oestrogen production.

Essential oils

A mixture of lavender, frankincense, clary sage and rose otto will increase energy levels and assist in relieving the pain. Use these oils in the bath and do ask your husband or partner to massage some into your back before bed. The oils can then soak into the system overnight. Essential oils for massage must be blended with a carrier oil such as almond or avocado.

Castor oil compresses

These are very effective for heavy or painful periods and endometriosis. In fact any inflammatory or toxic condition is helped by castor oil packs. Soak four layers of cotton cloth 30 to 20 cm (12 x 8 inches) in castor oil - just enough so that it does not run off. Warm this in a steamer, place it on the abdomen and cover with a piece of plastic or greaseproof paper. Lie down and rest a hot water bag on top. A towel over the bag will maintain the heat longer. Stay in this position for at least two hours - overnight if possible. Daily treatment is necessary in severe cases but, as symptoms improve, the frequency can be reduced.

If you are in a vicious cycle of pain and drugs, and fear coming off the drugs because you know you will feel even worse, do give this regime a try because it has been very successful with my patients. It is always a good idea to find an alternative health practitioner to encourage you on your pathway. In my practice I have consistently eradicated endometriosis with the outlined dietary regime, supplements and herbs. Before and after scans have provided my patients with proof. However I must stress that the detoxifying diet is very important.

5. Fibrocystic Breast Disease

This is also known as cystic mastitis and is usually associated with PMS. Sometimes the condition is characterised by pain or tenderness, but often it is painless. The problem occurs because the breast tissue is stimulated twice monthly; by oestrogen first and then progesterone, and this leads to considerable overactivity of the glands in some women. They develop multiple nodules which may cause great tenderness. This condition is always cyclical, but in time the cysts may remain all month causing discomfort.

Caffeine may need to be strictly avoided for it often causes over-production of fibrous tissue and cystic fluid. One controlled study indicated a 95% improvement in women omitting caffeine in the diet. If abstinence seems to have no effect, caffeine could be taken in moderation. Many studies have been carried out with fibrocystic breast disease and caffeine. There seems to be no middle ground in the results - removal of this substance from the diet is either reported as the wonder cure or it apparently fails to make any difference. A 1985 study of 2,300 women found no association, with caffeine and tender breasts. On the other hand, findings from another group involving over 600 women found a positive association especially in those who ingested over 500 mg of caffeine daily. However, the greatest effect was in the women whose breast changes were of a type associated with the increased risk of breast cancer. Another study which used a mammogram to detect differences in breast tissue before and after abstaining from caffeine found that, although the women felt a reduction in breast tenderness, there was no significant change in the tissue when viewed on mammogram. It is certainly worth giving up caffeine to determine its effect on you and in terms of general health it is also a very good idea.

Vitamin A appears to be very effective in reducing symptoms of breast pain. One study using 150,000 IU daily for three months had very positive results in a group of women who had failed to respond to caffeine withdrawal. Some patients had to drop out because of headaches due to the high levels of vitamin A. However all side effects were reversed very quickly once the vitamin intake was stopped. Half of the women experienced a 50% reduction in breast size and the effects lasted for eight months after the trial period ended. High dose beta carotene might have been a better way of treating fibrocystic breast disease as it is completely non-toxic. Anyone likely to become pregnant should not take over 2,000 IU of vitamin A on a daily basis.

Vitamin E normalises hormones and so has a positive effect. It also reduces FSH and LH when they are overstimulated - a common occurrence in fibrocystic conditions. The dose of this vitamin needs to be quite high to beneficially affect breast tenderness. A 1982 study involving 26 women resulted in total relief of cystic conditions in 10 of the group and considerable benefit for 12 of the remainder. Vitamin E 600 IU was given to these women for a period of eight weeks. Another study showed a correction in the oestrogen/progesterone ratio after two months on vitamin E 600 IU daily - the breast tenderness was reduced in line with the improved hormone balance.

Iodine is anti-inflammatory and prevents fibrous tissue formation. It is also necessary for the thyroid to function correctly.

Omega 6 fatty acid has proven itself in a great many trials in the form of evening primrose or borage oil. The latter contains double the amount of GLA in comparison with evening primrose oil so half the dosage is needed. GLA is converted on a chemical pathway in the body, to little tissue hormones called prostaglandin E_1 which have a controlling effect on hormones, the immune system, the cardiovascular system, the passage of nerve messages and the health of the skin, hair and nails. It is known to reduce the secretion of prolactin which is a cause of tender breasts. A study involving nearly 300 women with persistent severe breast pain found that half of the participants responded positively. It is my experience with patients, that several months of supplementation is necessary for real benefit. After all, it takes time for the hormone balance to shift using the tools of nature.

Bowel toxaemia is commonly associated with breast disease so it is really important to eradicate any tendency to constipation.

Look at your diet and take a supplement of live acidophilus to keep the gut environment healthy. When the bowel contains too high a proportion of unhealthy organisms, hormones are altered into toxic metabolites and carcinogens. Meat eaters have bacteria in the colon that are capable of making their own oestrogens which are then absorbed into the bloodstream where they add to the existing overload. A high fibre diet is also very important because it decreases the transit time of matter through the gut so that toxins are not so readily absorbed. A vegan diet is recommended in all menstrual problems where excessive oestrogen is the aggravating factor. Farmed meat contains hormones fed to the animal when it was growing and the resulting colon bacteria in the gut further increase the load. Vegetarian women excrete three times more unwanted oestrogen than meat eaters and do not have the problem of absorbing it from unfriendly bacteria.

Treatment

Diet

Vegan and high in fibre is the quickest dietary route for solving this condition. A little fish is the first animal protein to be reintroduced once symptoms improve.

Make sure that you get complete protein on a daily basis by combining whole grains and pulses. These both contain very high levels of fibre. The bulk of the diet should be fruit and vegetables, of which half should be raw.

Use sprouted seeds and pulses in your salads and start using seaweed as part of your daily diet. This contains high levels of iodine which is part of the cure. Try hijiki or arame first as they are easy to cook and do not have an unpleasant texture. They come in finely shredded form which requires soaking before boiling for about ten minutes. Add a little soy sauce and store in the refrigerator for use on your salads. Drink herbal teas in place of coffee and tea.

A juice fast, even a fruit and vegetable only diet, reduces symptoms markedly.

Avoid

Saturated fats in the form of meat and dairy products.

All processed oils, margarine and whipped up cooking fats and everything made from them. Use only extra virgin olive oil for all your cooking and salad dressings.

All caffeine, which means coffee, tea, chocolate and cola drinks.

All processed foods, which means white flour, white rice and sugar and everything made from them. Use food that has had minimal damage done by man!

Alcohol - an occasional glass of wine is of value to the spirit, but if it seems to have a negative effect then do without for a period.

Oral contraceptives.

Supplements of value

- **Potassium iodide** - 200 to 300 mcg or kelp tablets daily.
- **Vitamin B6** - 100 to 200 mg daily clears excess oestrogen and balances hormones. I always prescribe magnesium with this because a deficiency will reduce the effect of vitamin B6.
- **Vitamin B complex** - in low dose daily. This would be best in the form of a multivitamin/mineral which would also provide trace minerals like selenium and chromium.
- **Beta carotene** - 90 mg daily for several weeks and then reduce to 45 mg. If this amount makes your skin appear yellow, then take the equivalent in vitamin A instead, as this is not stored in the skin like beta carotene (but only if you are not likely to become pregnant).
- **Vitamin C** - 500 mg with **bioflavonoids** 250 mg - three times daily.
- **Vitamin E** - 600 IU with **selenium** 200 mcg daily.

- **Zinc** - 30 mg daily as citrate.
- **GLA as evening primrose oil** - 2000 mg daily - or as **borage oil** 1000 mg.
- **Flaxseed oil** - 3000 mg daily.
- **Potassium chloride** - 65 mg three times daily or use the tissue salt, kali chlor to reduce tissue congestion.
- **Acidophilus** - one capsule twice daily of a guaranteed live variety.

Herbs

These are chosen for their ability to increase the lymphatic drainage of the tissues and reduce the cystic formation. Useful herbs are:

Figwort, poke root, echinacea, red clover, plantain, burdock root and **thuja.** These may be mixed together in equal amounts in tincture form and the dose is half a teaspoon three times daily.

It is also a good idea to take a herb such as agnus castus for balancing the hormones. Buy tablets of these from a health food shop.

A few of my patients with a breast lump of unknown type have opted for a trial period on herbs and the above supplements before undergoing an invasive biopsy. This was always with their doctors' knowledge. In these cases I used the above treatment protocol along with the detoxifying Hoxey herbs against cancer and witnessed my patients' joy at seeing their lump steadily shrink. In the case of breast cancer, if you do choose surgery, statistics indicate a much higher success rate if it is carried out during the second half of the menstrual cycle. The rise of metastasis is increased with surgery during the first half of the cycle.

Homoeopathy

Dose with 6C potency three times daily. These remedies all fit the symptoms of tender or painful breasts premenstrually.

- **Iodum** - especially if there is a feeling of weakness during menses, a wedge-like pain in the ovaries or when the periods are irregular.
- **Calc. carb.** - especially if tired, feeling clumsy, inclined to cold sweats, craving sweet things, headaches before menses and cutting pains during.
- **Conium** - breasts hard and painful to touch. Periods painful with drawing pain down the thighs.
- **Pulsatilla** - especially if periods are irregular and you are inclined to burst into tears and need sympathy.
- **Lachesis** - everything is worse in the morning. The breasts feel inflamed and may be bluish. Every thing improves once the menstrual flow begins.
- **Nat. mur.** - particularly if the menses are irregular and profuse with bearing-down pains; fluid retention is also a feature and you may feel sad or irritable, but not respond to sympathy.

6. Ovarian Cyst

These fluid-filled sacs generally occur because of toxicity or hormonal imbalance. They cause symptoms only if they are large enough to press on other organs. They are a risk only if they become large enough to burst and possibly cause peritonitis. Cysts may also interfere with hormone production if they invade the ovarian tissue.

Treatment

A detoxification may be necessary, in which case follow the dietary recommendations in the chapter on endometriosis. Otherwise follow the general recommendations for diet and supplements in fibrocystic breast disease.

Herbs

The following herbs cleanse the blood, lymph and bowel, balance the hormones and tone the ovaries.

- **False unicorn** - to improve ovarian function and adjust the hormones.
- **Cramp bark** - for ovarian pain and an astringent effect.
- **Poke root** - for improving the lymph drainage from the ovaries.
- **Red clover** - for its tonic effect and its blood and lymph cleansing ability.
- **Yellow dock** - as a cleanser of the blood, liver and the bowel.
- **Golden seal** - for heavy, painful periods, as an antibacterial agent and for its tonic and astringent properties.

Mix these tinctures together and take one teaspoon twice daily or blend all the dried herbs in equal quantities and make a tea with 30 g (1 oz) to 500 ml of water. Drink one third twice daily. Alternatively, most of these herbs are available in various combinations from health food stores. It is also wise to take some agnus castus to assist in the hormone regulation.

Homeopathy

Dose with 6C potency three times daily. Constitutional therapy rather than the following symptomatic therapy is normally required.

- **Lachesis** - for left ovarian pain which is worse in the morning. All symptoms improve once the period starts.
- **Apis** - for stinging pain especially in the right ovary.
- **Colocynthis** - for small cysts which cause a boring pain through the abdomen. Doubling over relieves the pain to a certain extent.
- **Lilium tig** - right ovarian pain extending to the thighs.

7. Amenorrhoea

This is a complete absence of periods, which can have various causes. Finding the cause and treating it is the only way. However, at the same time the diet has to be optimal and herbs or homeopathic remedies may be used to speed a return to normal health.

Anorexia or excessive weight loss is a certain cause of amenorrhoea because of nutritional deficit. Any woman who eats very poorly on a long-term basis may also stop menstruating. Anaemia is another reason for this condition, as is a sluggish thyroid. This gland is partially responsible for clearing oestrogen through the liver so that the progesterone can be produced for the second half of the cycle. Excessive exercise will cause amenorrhoea - this is a problem for many female athletes who train too hard. Other common causes are coming off the pill and stress. The latter is a lifestyle problem and Part 1, chapter 19 will help you sort this out. Anorexia is a very complex condition to deal with. In my clinical experience, some young girls develop anorexic symptoms because of primary nutritional deficiencies and when these are replaced, normal feeding patterns return. I have even found the occasional case where an allergic reaction to a particular food disturbed the appetite centre in the brain so much that anorexic behaviour developed. The proof of these theories lies in the fact that a complete cure was incredibly rapid once the nutrition was corrected. So, before rushing off for months of counselling, give this possibility a thought. Teenagers whose menses are slow to come on stream, often have nutritional deficiencies, usually of zinc, magnesium and vitamin B6.

Treatment

Diet

This needs to be rich in nutrients which will keep the ovaries, thyroid and adrenal glands functioning well. Both the menopause and PMS diets are suitable. As PMS is not an issue when you do not get a monthly period, it is not necessary to eat between meals. It is only required for those who have low blood sugar problems.

When you eat fast food in restaurants and processed food from supermarkets, your stomach is easily satisfied, but your body is distressed because it receives no nutrients with which to function. The human body is an amazing piece of engineering and always endeavours to maintain all systems in spite of poor nutrition. However, eventually certain parts break down when they do not receive the necessities of life in the correct amounts.

Supplements of value

These are designed to balance hormones. You can often buy many of the nutrients in a single capsule .

- **Vitamin A** - 25,000 to 50,000 IU increases oestrogen or take 45-90 mg daily of beta carotene in preference if you hope to become pregnant.
- **Vitamin E** - 200 IU daily.
- **Multivitamin/mineral** - daily to supply B complex, selenium and zinc. High dose zinc may be necessary.
- **Vitamin B6** - 100 mg daily.
- **Magnesium** - 400 mg daily.
- **GLA** as **evening primrose oil** - 1000 mg daily or half the dose of **borage oil.**
- **Vitamin C** - 2,000 mg three times daily will often bring on a late period.

  Vitamin B12 - 1000 mcg daily in sublingual form regulates menses so this may be worth trying or, better still, a course of injections.

  Potassium chloride - 65 mg three times daily or the tissue salt, kali chlor.
- **Kelp** - or seaweed in the diet.

Herbs

- **Blue cohosh** - this is a very specific uterine tonic which combines well with false unicorn, motherwort and yarrow.

- **Black cohosh** - contracts the uterus and increases the menstrual flow. This herb is very useful in hormone imbalance and combines well with blue cohosh.
- **Motherwort** - tones the lining of the uterus and should be part of every blend of herbs for amenorrhoea. It promotes menstruation. It is also good for calming the mind.
- **Life root** - another good uterine tonic which stimulates menstruation and is highly recommended in cases of suppressed menses. It combines well with false unicorn and motherwort.
- **Southernwood** - tones the uterus and stimulates menstruation. It calms the nervous system and combines well with false unicorn in delayed menses.
- **False unicorn** - one of the best strengtheners of the reproductive system. It is a uterine tonic and menstrual stimulator which is especially useful in amenorrhoea.
- **Ginger** - improves the circulation to the uterine tissue and therefore the flow of nutrients. It is also a very effective promoter of menstruation.
- **Rue** - the leaves of this plant when taken as an infusion will bring on a late period. It combines well with false unicorn and life root.

Useful recipes

- Equal parts of Motherwort, false unicorn and life root.
- 3 parts motherwort, 2 parts chamomile and 1 part of each blue cohosh and ginger.

Mix these herbs in dried form (buy roots in powdered form) and drink one tea cup of infusion twice daily. Make the infusion with one teaspoon to a teacup of water. Tinctures are easier to handle. The dose is half to one teaspoon three times daily of a single herb or of a blend of several.

Essential oils

See chapter Part 1, chapter 8 on essential oils for the best way to use these healing agents.

- **Chamomile** - is wonderful for aches, pains, stresses and irritability, also for all menstrual problems including amenorrhoea.
- **Clary sage** - is a nerve tonic for nervous types and is also a uterine tonic. Clary is the best oil for depression and is also excellent in panicky states.
- **Hyssop** - is a tonic for any system which is in a weakened state, but should be avoided in pregnancy.
- **Juniper** - has a sedative effect as well as the well-known diuretic action. It is also used in amenorrhoea as it induces menstruation.

Homoeopathy

Dose 30C daily for one month.

- **Nat. mur.** - a primary remedy for amenorrhoea which is particularly relevant where long-term stress is a factor or there has been a recent emotional shock which triggered the loss of menses. This woman is inclined to be solitary, tired nervous.
- **Aconite** - for when periods stop suddenly, due to great emotional shock or exposure to cold. Vagina may be dry, hot and sensitive.
- **Dulcamara** - periods stop after being very cold. The suppression is due to cold or dampness.
- **Calcarea** - for when there is PMS but no period arrives. This woman is tired and chilly. Her legs feel very heavy. She is inclined to be flabby, overweight, sensitive to cold and she perspires heavily.

- **Lycopodium** - periods are disrupted by even slight emotional upset. Other symptoms may include abdominal pain, digestive upsets, headaches and feeling faint.
- **Pulsatilla** - for periods that are irregular and changeable. Pain in the back and feeling tired. This woman likes to be out in the fresh air. She is inclined to weepiness and (unlike the Nat. mur. woman) likes to be comforted.

Irregular periods

This is a sign of hormonal imbalance which, like amenorrhoea, can have a variety of causes. As with other conditions in this book, the diet has to be corrected and supplements taken to regulate the hormones. Taking herbs in addition, will speed the process of normalisation. Essential oils are a slower but a very pleasant way of doing the same thing. Take the supplements from those listed under Amenorrhoea along with hormone balancing herbs such as agnus castus and dong quai. If your periods just happen to be late each month but are fairly regular, then rue tea taken four hourly for a few days before the due date will probably sort out the problem. It can be combined with false unicorn and life root. Southernwood would be another good choice.

A naturopath or medical herbalist can best guide you in the choice of herbs.

8. Infertility

This can have a multitude of causes, from hormonal imbalance to nutritional deficiency, and some have damaged reproductive systems because of previous infections and scarring. *Emotional trauma at any stage of life can also prevent conception.*

If you have been unable to become pregnant in spite of many months of unprotected sex, first get yourself checked out for any physical impediments such as a retroverted uterus, blocked tubes, ovarian cysts or endometriosis. If all is well, then you need to consider emotions, stress, toxic body conditions and nutritional deficiencies in relationship with a hormone imbalance. The heavy-duty hormone therapy really should be the last resort.

Where conception occurs but is followed by immediate miscarriage, this is probably due to nutritional deficiencies like zinc or vitamin E. This may also occur as a result of toxic accumulations from smoking, drinking alcohol and coffee or eating too much processed foods.

Essentials for conception

Pregnancy requires a follicle stimulating hormone (FSH) for the initial growth and development in the ovaries and the luteinizing hormone (LH) to further develop the ovarian follicles and promote ovulation. Both these hormones are required for the secretion of oestrogen. The LH also promotes progesterone release. Oestrogen builds up the lining in the uterus to receive a fertilised ovum and progesterone maintains the pregnancy, along with placental hormones. A healthy body with all nutrients present is a basic necessity for normal hormonal function.

Vitamin B6 and magnesium are needed for the pituitary to secrete the hormones FSH and LH. Vitamin E assists reproduction by normalising oestrogen. There was a very interesting study in 1979 of infertile women who also suffered PMS. These women were given 100 to 800 mg of vitamin B6 daily for at least six months. The amount taken was determined by what was required to alleviate the symptoms of PMS. Eleven of the fourteen women conceived within six months and one at eleven months.

Vitamin B12 and folic acid deficiencies are also causes of infertility so these should be in a multivitamin in adequate amounts.

GLA as evening primrose or **borage oil** leads to formation of tiny tissue hormones called PGE_1 which regulate sex hormones. For these to function correctly it is important to avoid all processed oils and margarines, sugar and white flour and limit saturated fat. Eat a few mixed raw seeds daily with the breakfast fruit and yoghurt. Walnuts, pumpkin, sunflower and sesame seeds contain the precursors of GLA.

Omega 3 oils in the form of flax and pumpkin seeds, soya beans and oily fish are also vital for reproduction.

Zinc is essential for the production of the pituitary hormone, which then stimulates the secretion of the sex hormones from the ovaries. It is also involved in the growth of the sexual organs as well as activation of the thyroid hormone.

Iron deficiency will cause infertility so check both your haemoglobin and ferritin levels and, if it is necessary to take supplements, do so separately from zinc.

The amino acid **cysteine** is especially high in FSH and LH but it requires as co-factors vitamin C, E, folic acid, B6 and the minerals selenium and magnesium. Without these, cysteine activity is reduced.

Vitamin C replenishes the ovaries and has been known to work where Clomid has failed!

The thyroid gland plays a part in stimulating ovulation and if a condition of subclinical hypothyroidism exists, the gland needs to be stimulated to normal function. Do this with exercise, and nutrients such as B vitamins, iodine, phenylalanine or tyrosine and magnesium. Some times thyroxine is being produced in adequate amounts but a lack of zinc means that it is not being activated. A sluggish thyroid will not show up on blood tests, but it can still inhibit conception.

Potassium chloride is essential for proper ovarian function and **vitamin A** keeps the cilia moving in the Fallopian tubes. I have known two infertile women to become pregnant after taking potassium chloride with a multivitamin.

The Australian bushflower remedy **'she oak'** is often used successfully to clear emotional blocks to conception.

Treatment

Diet

Largely vegetarian with a little fish and egg. The polyunsaturated fats in the form of seeds and oily fish are essential. It is just as important to avoid all processed oils and strictly curtail white flour and sugar products as these block the activity of the natural oils.

Avoid

Caffeine.

Rutin - a bioflavonoid which is used as a contraceptive[1] to prevent the fertilisation of ova. This is found in buckwheat, elder berry and in many vitamin C products but it is only necessary to avoid Rutin in supplement form.

High animal protein diets and processed foods.

Toxic conditions from a poor diet and lack of exercise. If toxins are not eliminated from the mucous membranes, an allergic reaction can occur between the sperm and the cervix. In this case a juice fast is needed to properly detoxify the tissues.

Supplements of value

- A quality **natural multivitamin/mineral** tablet daily to include all the B's and selenium. Folic acid should be 400 to 800 mcg and a course of B12 injections may be useful.
- **Vitamin B6** - 50 mg twice daily, although considerably higher doses may be necessary.

1 Papaya fruit is also known in Asia as an effective contraceptive.

- **Vitamin E** - 1,000 IU daily.
- **Zinc** - 30 mg daily as citrate or amino acid chelate.
- **Magnesium** - 500 mg daily with **calcium** 500 to 1000 mg.
- **Vitamin C** - 1 g four times daily.
- **Evening primrose oil** - 500 mg four to six times daily or half the amount of **borage oil**.
- **Beta carotene** - 15 mg daily.
- **Cysteine and Phenylalanine** - 250 mg each twice daily with juice half an hour before meals.
- **Potassium chloride** - 65 to 100 mg three times daily.
- **She oak** - 7 drops of the dilute flower remedy twice daily.

Read the chapter on stress and use the appropriate oils such as germanium, rosemary, clary sage, fennel and basil.

Herbs

The following herbs are chosen for their ability to tone the uterus and balance the hormones; both of which is necessary for a successful conception.

Dong quai - increases the circulation to the reproductive organs which has a toning effect. It promotes fertility and can be bought in Chinese medicine stores in tablet form combined with other herbs. Danggui should not be taken separately. Chinese herbalists always recommend this herb in combination with others. This herb is not to be continued once the first period is missed.

Red raspberry leaves - are a universal uterine tonic and also used in pregnancy to tone the uterus. It does not cause contractions, but once the uterus does start contracting, raspberry leaf makes the uterus work more effectively. Buy as tablets or make an infusion from the herb and drink three cups daily.

Red clover flowers - are a blood and uterine tonic par excellence. This herb balances the pH of the tissues, including the birth canal, and contains a very extensive range of vitamins and minerals. Red clover makes a pleasant tea and would combine well with nettles, which is another uterine tonic with hormone-balancing properties.

False unicorn - is a major hormone adjuster and uterine tonic. It promotes fertility and prevents threatened miscarriage, but is not used throughout a pregnancy - only as a fertility promoter.

Homeopathy

Folliculinum - 30C monthly for those who cannot get pregnant after coming off the pill, and where the periods are irregular after coming off the pill.

Agnus castus - 6C twice daily until ten days before the period if pituitary function is poor.

Sabina - 30C monthly if prone to miscarriage before twelve weeks.

Constitutional treatment is important.

Male infertility

In the last fifty years the average sperm count in Western countries has dropped by 30 to 40%. A major reason for infertility appears to be environmental poisons. This means smoking, drugs and alcohol, pesticides, computer screens, microwaves and a variety of electro-magnetic horrors which have become part of modern life. An interesting study reported in Denmark revealed that organic farmers had double the sperm levels of greenhouse workers. The latter are exposed to very concentrated levels of pesticides in a closed environment. Infertile men would be wise to be tested for tissue levels of heavy metals and pesticides in case this is the reason for the low sperm counts. These can be removed from the body with nutritional and homeopathic remedies. In fact, detoxifying and correcting the nutritional base is the only sensible way to resolve infertility.

In this age of eating fast food and relying on the processed produce found in supermarkets, the human species is seriously depleted in unprocessed polyunsaturated fats. One of the many downsides of this is in the area of fertility. Without a proper balance of omega 3 and 6 oils in the diet, production and motility of sperm is reduced. Processed food is loaded with omega 6 oil, but it is in toxic trans form, which is not only useless to the human body, but actually elbows out the essential natural forms of this oil. It is important to turn back to using olive oil or a little saturated fat for cooking and eating polyunsaturated oils in the form of walnuts, seeds (flax, sunflower, sesame and pumpkin), soya beans and oily fish. Salmon, sardines mackerel or herrings should be eaten three times a week for good health and increased fertility.

Men who have low sperm counts often lack two amino acids which are formed from arginine. Studies using arginine indicate success in increasing sperm count as long as the initial level was not below 20 million per millilitre. The effective dose was 4 g grams daily.

A study using 3 g daily of the amino acid l-carnitine on infertile men resulted in 79% responding with a mean increase in sperm count from 88 million to 159 million per millilitre and the amount of mobile sperm increased 100%. The actual mobility rose by 50%.

Zinc is an essential mineral for proper sperm levels and motility. One study showed an improved sperm count after four months of elemental zinc supplementation of 60 mg daily. Another group of 37 males with sperm counts below 25 million were given the same amount of zinc for six weeks. There was a significant increase in sperm counts of those who initially had low testosterone, but in the men with normal hormone levels, the sperm levels were unchanged by the zinc. Low levels of zinc allow toxic chemicals to take root in the body and this leads to further depletion of zinc.

Vitamin C protects against oxidative attacks on sperm. It is also known to increase sperm count, the motility and reduce agglutination. In a study of 35 men with varying degrees of sperm agglutination, 500 mg vitamin C was given twice daily for three weeks and the percentage of agglutinated sperm was reduced markedly.

Vitamin B12 may be useful in some cases. Even without a deficiency of this vitamin, many conditions will improve after a course of injections. This also applies to low sperm count. One study indicated that even those with a count below 20 million per millilitre could improve after daily injections of 1500 to 6000 mcg.

Selenium deficiency leads to reduced sperm motility and this can be increased 100% with regular supplementation.

Co-enzyme Q10 is another antioxidant which also plays a role in increasing the motility and number of sperm in infertile men.

Supplements of value

- **Arginine** - 2 g twice daily for sperm production and motility.
- **Methionine** - 500 mg twice daily as a co-factor to arginine.
- **Carnitine** - 1.5 g twice daily for sperm motility.

Take these three amino acids with juice 30 to 60 minutes before food.

- **Co-enzyme Q10** - 50 mg daily.
- **Omega 3 oil** as flaxseed oil or EPA/DHA from fish oil.
- **Omega 6 oil** as borage or evening primrose oil.
- **Selenium** - 200 mcg daily.
- **Zinc** - 30 mg twice daily.
- **Manganese** - 10 mg daily as it works with zinc.
- **Vitamin C** - 1 g twice daily.
- **Potassium chloride** - 65 mg three times daily or the tissue salt kali chlor.
- **Vitamin B12 injections** - oral doses are very poorly absorbed.

9. Candida Albicans

This is a fungus which is present inside everyone. It normally inhabits the bowel and does no harm as it is kept in control by the immune system and the normal healthy intestinal micro-organisms. However, when the immune system is damaged and the microflora wiped out by antibiotics or other drugs, the candida is no longer held in check and so proliferates. The speed at which this happens depends on the health of the person and his diet. If the latter contains processed foods, alcohol, sugar and white flour, candida will spread rapidly because it just loves junk food.

Eventually the fungus changes shape into a form which puts down roots into the intestinal wall. This makes the intestines too porous and allows partially digested food, fungus, parasites and toxins to readily pass into the bloodstream. The immune system then recognises them as foreign and an allergic reaction occurs. Once the candida has penetrated the colon wall, it can spread to any part of the body via the bloodstream and cause havoc to its human host with a variety of unpleasant symptoms. If it becomes established in the lymphatic system, the fungus can recolonise the bowel at will. This means that treatment of the bowel only can be self-defeating - the whole body must be cleansed. An added insult is that the body becomes sensitised to all other forms of fungus and a wide variety of even natural foods must be avoided quite aside from the simple carbohydrate on which candida lives. By this time a person feels exhausted to say the least, if not 'sick all over'.

Candida of the vagina has increased dramatically in the past decade until it now seems to be one of the most common causes of discharge. A study in the 1970's found that all cases also had a proliferation of candida in the intestines. The contraceptive pill, antibiotics, steroids and a junk food diet are all heavily implicated in causing this condition. Furthermore, research has highlighted a very sinister side of candida overgrowth. It has become clear that if a staphylococcus infection occurs simultaneously, the bacteria take on a high-powered virulence against which antibiotics have no effect; cases of toxic shock syndrome have resulted.

Diagnosis

Because we all have candida inside us, laboratory tests are of little value in diagnosing systemic infestation. Rather the total symptom picture is important. The following are symptoms of candida, but a person needs to have several at one time before a diagnosis is positive as other conditions such as post-viral fatigue syndrome can also cause some of these symptoms.

Intestinal bloating and flatulence, nausea, abdominal pain, diarrhoea or constipation. All of these symptoms are worse after eating sugar or refined carbohydrate.

Vaginal thrush, persistent itch or burning, menstrual disturbances, endometriosis, PMS, recurrent cystitis or urethritis.

Depression, fuzzy headedness, poor memory and concentration, fatigue, dizziness, mood swings, confusion, anxiety, headaches, irritability or erratic vision.

Itchy nose, oral thrush, pains and tightness in the chest, sore throats, bad breath, nasal congestion or a post-nasal drip.

Aches and pains in muscles unrelated to exercise, tingling, joint swelling, numbness or burning sensations.

Feeling unwell in damp or mouldy conditions and reacting strongly to chemicals, perfumes, fumes, synthetics or tobacco smoke.

Athlete's foot, rashes or fungal patches on the skin.

Multiple allergies and cravings for sugar, alcohol and bread.

The symptoms depend on which part of the body has been infiltrated by the candida. In addition to several of the above conditions being persistent, there should be a history of one of the following: The taking of antibiotics, either for a month at a time or a few short courses within the past year. Use of the contraceptive pill for over one year. A short course of cortisone-type drugs.

Treatment

There is no point in treating candida at a local level and ignoring the systemic aspect. Using antifungals for a vaginal infestation and not treating the gut just ensures repeated attacks and in the long run there is a risk of the whole body becoming affected.

Some people suffer greatly from candida - in fact, some people's lives are completely disabled by it. The condition is easy to treat if done in a logical sequence, but results take time. Even when symptoms disappear, a very long period of dietary restriction is essential while the bowel wall heals and once again becomes a barrier against fungus and toxins. In serious illness, the adrenal glands will be stressed and the immune system severely weakened. Unless both systems are strengthened the antifungal/antiparasitic treatment will not hold for long.

Treatment outline

Starve the fungus.

Destroy it.

Destroy any parasites which are probably also present in the intestines and perhaps the lymphatics.

Strengthen the immune system and liver function so that they can destroy the candida and detoxify the body. No one develops candida unless the immune system has first been damaged.

Ensure a healthy intestinal environment.

Heal the bowel wall.

Diet

High fibre, high complex carbohydrate, moderate protein and low fat.

Abundant vegetables twice daily especially asparagus, broccoli, beetroot, cabbage, peppers, onions, garlic and cucumber.

Juiced vegetables daily, as the diet must be 75% alkaline forming to inhibit fungus.

Fruit in moderation. It is seldom necessary to avoid fruit but eat it whole and not juiced. Avoid very low fibre fruit like melon and very sweet fruits like grapes, dried fruit and bananas until well on the road to recovery.

Live plain yoghurt in moderation.

Whole grains such as oats, millet and rice to be used liberally. Toasted 100% black rye bread is all right in moderation but restrict wheat as the carbohydrate ferments easily.

Pulses, lentils, chickpeas, soya beans, pinto beans etc.,

Sprouted peas, beans, seeds and grains, especially mung and alfalfa.

All seeds, plus almonds, walnuts, fresh coconut and buckwheat.

Oily fish and white fish, egg and low-fat cottage cheese, meat in moderation, but only if free of hormones and anti-biotics.

Lamb and organic chicken or wild game are the safest.

Two teaspoons of extra virgin olive oil daily, as a dressing.

Herbal tea, mineral water, vegetable juices and broth as drinks. Take 1 litre (two pints) daily.

Cinnamon, thyme, lemon balm, rosemary, oregano and garlic are destructive to candida.

All food should be organic and as much raw as possible.

Avoid

Chemicals such as birth control pills, antibiotics, cortisone, preservatives, colourings, flavourings, perfumes, fumes, MSG, and chemical cleaning products.

All sugar, white flour, white rice and everything made from them, e.g. jams, pickles, frozen and canned vegetables, cakes, biscuits, crackers, pasta, pizza and processed breakfast cereals. Even healthy sweeteners will feed candida, so avoid maple, corn and rice bran syrups and honey, as well as sucrose, dextrose, glucose, fructose, lactose, maltose, galactose, molasses, mannitol and sorbitol.

All refined, canned, processed and packaged food, as sugar or yeast is often involved.

Alcohol, tea and coffee as they stimulate the release of sugar from the liver.

All carbonated drinks, squashes, fruit juices, dried fruit, bananas and sweet grapes.

All malted products including cereals and malted milk, etc.

Milk because of the milk sugar content.

Meat that is not organic, as the antibiotics and hormone residues will increase the candida growth.

Processed meats including salami, sausage, hamburgers and bacon.

Foods to which you are allergic.

Oils, except guaranteed cold-pressed polyunsaturates and olive oil, otherwise the immune response to the candida is inhibited.

Microwave cooking, as enzymes are inhibited and the molecular structure of foods altered.

The above restrictions may be enough for conditions where the symptoms are not too severe. However for some it is vital that they also avoid the following three groups of ferments, moulds and yeasts. No yeast or mould will feed candida, but when a person is heavily infested with this fungus, she can become sensitised to all other forms, in that they make her feel very unwell and slow the recovery. A good rule of thumb would be to avoid them until feeling much improved on the treatment and then experiment with widening your food choices by first adding cooked mushrooms, bread and marmite. If all is well, try the ferments like tofu and vinegar. You will soon know if something has to be removed from your diet for a further period as your bloating, fatigue or mood swings will increase. Those who have serious fungal conditions may have to avoid the following foods for as long as six months while others may be able to reintroduce them in a few weeks.

Fermentation foods are tofu, soya sauce, vinegar and everything made from them; dressings, mayonnaise, pickles and smoked foods like salmon and corned beef; sauces, alcohol and Indian or Chinese tea except green tea.

Moulds are present on leftover food, dried fruit, and all peanuts and any other nuts that are not fresh, mouldy cheese, mushrooms; and in damp basements, mouldy bathrooms and cupboards and on rugs. Even some herbal teas may be mouldy so buy herbs from reliable medicinal suppliers.

Yeasts are found in bread, pizza, commercial cakes, biscuits, crackers and bread-crumbed food, Brewer's yeast, marmite and vegemite. Some vitamins and minerals are not guaranteed yeast free. Beer, cider, wines and malted drinks contain yeasts. For those who wonder if there is anything they can eat, here are some menu ideas.

Breakfast

Raw muesli which is sugar and fruit free. Add chopped fresh nuts and seeds, fresh coconut and wheatgerm.

Oatmeal, millet, brown rice or buckwheat porridge. Serve all cereals with sugar-free soya milk, nut milk or live plain yoghurt.

Cooked eggs and yeast free bread, wholegrain Ryvita or rice cakes.

Wholewheat or buckwheat pancakes with butter or sugar-free jam and yoghurt.

Lunch

A herbal or Spanish omelette.

Low-fat cottage cheese.

Add a baked potato with a yoghurt dressing that has lemon juice added.

Dishes made from dried peas and beans.

Dahl made from lentils and spices.

Salads made from brown rice, wholegrain pasta, buckwheat, barley or millet, with added flavourings like yoghurt and horse-radish or garlic, oil and lemon juice. Add chopped vegetables to this or stir in curried vegetables.

Home-made soups with vegetables, beans or grains.

Nut roasts or patties.

Any of the choices for lunch should be served with a large salad and sprouted peas, beans or seeds. Dressings are made of extra virgin olive oil, lemon juice, garlic and herbs.

Dinner

Fish, especially salmon, mackerel, sardines or trout.

Lamb or genuine free-range poultry.

Lamb's liver or kidney.

Vegetarian protein as at lunch. If not eating animal protein be sure to combine beans and grains or nuts/seeds in the same day to make complete protein.

The above suggestions should accompany a large plate of vegetables lightly steamed or as a salad. Use a great variety of vegetables every day.

If eating out, starters could be salads or plain asparagus; the main course, fresh salmon and vegetables; and the dessert, fresh fruit once it is again permitted. Remember: no roasting or frying. Wash all fruit and vegetables thoroughly as they often have mould on them. Yeast will grow on stale grains and nuts; pistachios grow it particularly easily. The peanut crops in the world are infested with a toxic mould so no one should eat them. The amount of raw vegetables eaten would depend on the your digestive system. You may need to slowly increase the amount, rather than suddenly start eating large servings.

Snacks

Raw vegetable sticks, seeds (pumpkin, sesame, sunflower and linseed), yoghurt and herbal tea or mineral water.

The above dietary program starves the fungus so that it begins to die off.

Supplements of value - adult doses

Antifungal

- **L.acidophilus** and **bifido bacteria** in capsule form or as a powder. The product must be guaranteed potent, require refrigeration and have an expiry date. It repopulates the bowel with healthy bacteria, makes the B vitamin biotin and controls the fungus.

- **Fructo-oligosaccharides** (FOS) - one tablespoon or more daily, as this product encourages the healthy bacteria to recolonise in the intestines. It can also be used as a sweetener as it does not feed candida. FOS is found naturally in the fibre of fruit and vegetables.
- **Biotin** - 400 mcg daily, and two teaspoons of olive oil daily. Both of these prevent the candida from changing to the invasive form. Excessive biotin has the opposite effect.
- **Garlic** - 1 to 2 g three times daily, raw or the equivalent in dried form. One very large clove weighs 5 to 6 g.
- **Aloe vera** juice - two tablespoons daily.
- **Fibre** as guar gum, psyllium or flaxseeds - one tablespoon at night to flush toxins from the colon.
- **Betaine hydrochloric acid** tablets and digestive enzymes with meals to increase stomach acidity and prevent the fungus spreading upwards. The enzymes ensure complete digestion of food.
- **Bromelain** - 500 mg three times daily with meals to clear away intestinal mucus which shelters parasites.

The following should be added after an initial period of starving the candida through dietary control. Depending on the severity of the condition, one or more would be used for about two months.

- **Caprylic acid, Mycopryl** or **Mycocidin** - in capsule form according to the manufacturer's instructions. Usually the dose is gradually increased to reduce die-off symptoms which worsen conditions like fuzzy heads. The capricin and mycopryl are coconut derivatives which go through the gut destroying yeast. The mycocidin is very similar to caprylic acid, but is extracted from castor bean oil and this also effectively destroys fungus.

- **Citricidal** (grapefruit seed extract) - according to manufacturer's instructions. This also destroys acidophilus, so extra needs to be taken whilst using this product.
- **Licorice, golden seal, walnut leaves, fennel, barberry** and **echinacea** - mix this herbal blend in equal weights and make a tea of 30 g (1 oz) to 500 ml of water and drink one third three times daily. Alternatively, find them in capsule form or make a tincture from the blend and take one teaspoon three times daily.
- **Pau d'arco** - 20 g to 500 ml and simmer for five minutes. Infuse another ten minutes and drink this tea in one day.
- **Tea tree** or **German chamomile oil** - 1 to 3 drops three times daily, orally.
- **Oregano** and **rosemary oil** extracts - in capsule form according to manufacturers instructions.
- **Walnut leaves** or **black walnut husks, artemisia annua** and **yerba santa** are all anti-parasitic herbs, but it is better to rid parasites under professional care where the dosage will be given according to individual requirement. Parasitic infestations are often present in those with candida because the unhealthy intestinal environment allows the growth of parasites as well as fungus.

Immune system support

Look for a supplement designed for immune system repair. It will supply the first eight supplements listed in similar amounts in a full day's dosage and possibly some herbs as well. These nutrients will also restore tired adrenal glands, but in that case, add 500 mg pantothenic acid and ginseng tea.

- **Beta carotene** - 6 mg or vitamin A 10,000 IU daily.
- **Vitamin C** - 500 mg three times daily.
- **Vitamin E** - 200 to 400 IU daily.
- **Vitamin B complex** - 25 to 50 mg daily.

- **Selenium** - 200 mcg daily.
- **Zinc** - 30 mg daily.
- **Manganese** - 5 mg daily.
- **GLA** as **evening primrose** oil - 2000 mg daily or half dose **borage** oil.
- A **calcium/magnesium** supplement supplying 250 mg of each daily.

Liver Support

This is important, as the liver has to detoxify the candida.

- **Lemon juice** in water or green vegetable juice daily before food, increases liver function.
- **Silymarin** herbal extract - 50 mg three times daily regenerates the liver and powerfully protects it.
- **Dandelion root** tea improves liver function, as do the barberry and golden seal herbs used to destroy candida.
- **Molybdenum** is necessary for forming the liver detoxifying enzymes, and will often clear the debilitating brain symptoms of confusion, poor concentration and fuzzy feelings.

Heal the bowel wall

This is vital so that the colon ceases to be porous to fungus and foods that are not properly digested. The acidophilus has some effect of course, together with the zinc, pantothenic acid (vitamin B5), folic acid and vitamin A, already indicated for immune competence.

Glucosamine (as NAG), 500 mg three times daily, holds together the cells lining the intestinal tract to reduce porosity. Butyric acid, 750 mg three times daily, provides the energy for the growth of the intestinal cells and is necessary for the adherence of healthy bacteria to the gut wall. Both of these products should be taken once the candida has been largely eliminated. Rice bran oil (gamma-oryzanol) will also soothe and heal an inflamed gut lining.

If the digestion is poor, it is wise to take digestive enzymes after meals and to drink peppermint tea. Where protein foods such as fish, meat and eggs tend to sit heavily in the stomach, a supplement of betaine hydrochloric acid taken before food will assist in the initial breakdown of protein so that the enzymes can digest these foods.

It is possible for symptoms to clear reasonably quickly with the above treatment and this tempts people to relax the diet. It is very important to resist, as the condition will only recur until the fungus is under complete control, the immune system is doing a good job of surveillance and the bowel has healed and been repopulated with the correct micro-organisms. In extreme cases this takes as long as two years. For those with less severe conditions, control may be possible with diet alone, although a general immune supplement and lactobacillus is advisable.

10. Vaginitis

Vaginal infections are one of the most common conditions in young women. This is probably due to a mixture of being sexually active, taking the contraceptive pill, and eating an inadequate diet that is nutritionally deficient.

Vaginitis needs to be taken seriously, as it may be associated with a chronic inflammation of the cervix or a sexually transmitted disease. If not treated adequately, infection can spread into the uterus and Fallopian tubes, causing endometriosis, salpingitis or pelvic inflammatory disease. Some women have a discharge at various times during the menstrual cycle which is caused by hormonal stimulation, but inflammation is not involved here and treatment is unnecessary.

Predisposing factors

If the pH of the vagina is changed, infection can readily develop. The 'pill' and a diet containing white flour products and sugar will make the vagina too alkaline. The healthy microflora which normally inhabit the vagina are also important because without them, mucus secretion is increased and this provides a fertile breeding ground for organisms. If the immune system is strong, infection is prevented. However, immune function is readily inhibited by a poor diet, the 'pill' and other drugs, unhealthy lifestyles, stress, illness and allergies.

Candida albicans (monilia)

This is by far the most common reason for vaginitis. It causes itching or burning and may be so thick that it looks like cottage cheese. Sometimes it appears as small white patches with a red border of inflamed tissue.

The increased use of the contraceptive pill, antibiotics and a poor diet cause the fungus to proliferate and treating only the local symptoms ensures constant recurrence of the condition. If candida is present in the vagina it is also flourishing in the gut, so a general systemic anti-candida treatment is required as well as ensuring that any existing predisposing factors are removed.

Topical treatment choices

Betadine, citricidal or **tea tree oil** douches daily for 2 to 3 weeks at a time. Add a garlic capsule to the solution.

Boric acid 600 mg put into capsules and inserted nightly for seven doses is a very effective treatment or make a solution with a little water and soak a tampon which is already inserted.

Two **L. acidophilus** capsules should be inserted nightly once the boric acid treatment is finished. Use a concentrated solution if it is easier.

Studies indicate that the herb **echinacea** will prevent the recurrence of vaginal candida in those who are frequently affected. Take it orally.

Marigold and **golden seal** herbs are healing and soothing as a douche.

Trichomonas

This is a sexually transmitted protozoa which may be found in the vagina, urethra and surrounding glands. It causes itching and burning and there is a frothy yellow/green discharge, sometimes with a fishy odour. It is often associated with gonorrhoea and is a major cause of cervical erosion. It is one of the reasons for the high rate of false positive cervical smears.

Treatment

Stimulate the immune system with a diet of whole natural foods, an abundance of fruit and vegetables and avoidance of sugar, white flour and all refined packaged food.

Avoid the contraceptive pill and other drugs.

Practise safe sex. Take the following natural supplements to strengthen the immune system, destroy the infection and improve the vaginal environment.

Supplements

- **Beta carotene** - 15 mg daily for a healthy vaginal lining resistant to infection.
- **Vitamin C** - 1 g four times daily.
- **Vitamin E** - 200 IU daily.
- **Selenium** - 100 mcg daily.
- **Zinc** - 15 to 25 mg daily as citrate.
- **B complex** - 50 mg daily.
- **Garlic** - 1 g three times daily.
- **L. acidophilus** - two capsules daily of a guaranteed potent type.
- **Glucosamine** (as NAG) - 1 g twice daily to quickly restore the normality of cells and fluids lining the vagina.

Herbs

- **Golden seal** - 0.5 g three times daily.
- **Echinacea** - 1 g three times daily.

These can also be made into a decoction and used as a douche.

Topical treatment

Insert two **L. acidophilus** capsules nightly or use a live yoghurt and choose from the following for douching twice daily for two to three weeks.

Tea tree oil, **peppermint** oil or **lavender** oil. Use 2.5 ml of one of these essential oils to 250 ml of water.

Betadine douche.

Zinc sulphate - 2% as a douche. Use one tablespoon to 500 ml of water.

Tampons may be inserted and then soaked in douche solutions with garlic added. Kyolic garlic is good and therefore effective as well as odourless. In the case of the essential oils, 1 to 5 % solutions may be used on a tampon twice weekly all day. Add squeezed garlic or garlic powder to all douching solutions as it is effective against all infecting agents in vaginitis; added chlorophyll is also very soothing.

Chlamydia

This genital infection is sexually transmitted and often associated with urethritis and inflammation of the cervix or Fallopian tubes in women. In men there may be proctitis or epididymitis.

Chlamydia is a parasitic bacterium which usually infects the cervix in women and the urethra of men and is often asymptomatic. Any discharge is like a thick mucus and there may be some burning on passing urine. The eyes and respiratory tract can be infected with chlamydia and, in the case of newborn infants from infected mothers, the eyes must be carefully treated immediately. Treatment should be vigorous as there is a risk of pelvic inflammatory disease, tubal scarring and infertility. Antibiotics may be needed as well as the herbs, but studies have shown that recurrence is more common in those taking antibiotics alone.

Because chlamydia tends to be symptom free, it is one of the most potentially harmful sexually transmitted diseases. This is because it is often detected only after pelvic inflammatory disease or sterility already exists. Chlamydia can remain undetected in cells for years and passed to any sexual partner during that time. When the immune system is weakened or a woman undergoes gynaecological surgery (including IUD insertion), the bacteria can spread to the uterus and Fallopian tubes. Anyone at risk should have regular checks so that treatment can be instigated early.

Treatment

Herbs

Use the same supplements as in trichomonas.

Golden seal, barberry and oregon (berberines). Mix these together in equal proportions and take 1 g of the powdered root, or one teaspoon of tincture three times daily.

Topical

Douche with **betadine** or 2% **zinc sulphate** solution twice daily and **berberine** tea once daily.

Add 2 drops of **Lugol's** solution and **garlic** to a daily **tea tree** oil douche.

Gardnerella

This is sometimes asymptomatic, but often the discharge has a foul odour. The treatment is the same as for chlamydia.

Homeopathy

For any of the infections. Dose 6C 4 to 6 times daily for ten days.

- **Borax** - an egg white discharge which irritates or itches.
- **Kreosotum** - milky discharge which is corrosive, burning or itchy. Pain in the lower back and great weakness.
- **Alumina** - chronic copious yellow discharge which hardens on underwear. Itching which is better for washing in cold water.
- **Bovista** - thick green discharge especially after periods.
- **Carbo veg.** - green discharge which burns, especially before periods.
- **Nit. ac.** - stitching pain in the vagina, flesh-coloured watery, smelly discharge.

- ***Mercurius*** - a foul smelling green discharge which burns or itches. Better for washing with cold water. Pain in the ovaries. Person sweats easily and may have bad breath.
- **Sepia** - yellow/green discharge and a stitching pain in the uterus. Itching worse when walking.

11. Cystitis

Cystitis is an inflammation of the bladder which is more common in women than men because the short urethra allows easy access for bacterial invasion. The usual infecting organisms are E.coli from the bowel or staphylococcus. Both bacteria can be cleared with herbs or homeopathic remedies so there is usually no need for antibiotics which will only increase the risk of thrush. In some cases there is no infection because the symptoms are produced by a low fluid intake, resulting in a very concentrated urine causing the irritation. Other common non-infective causes of cystitis are nylon underwear, chlorinated swimming pools and bubble baths.

A chronic inflammation of the urethra or bladder may occur in a very tense, anxious individual. The symptoms are fierce and debilitating, strike at random and may last for weeks. Deep-acting homeopathy is the only way to cure this condition. A chronic inflammation may also occur as the result of the pill, antibiotics or from a food allergy. Short sharp attacks can be due to intercourse.

The elderly are sometimes prone to a low grade cystitis where pain is not severe but a constant desire to pass urine is present. This is normally a catarrhal condition which can be cleared by increasing fluid and taking the tissue salt kali chlor. A herbal tea of marshmallow, golden rod, eyebright and buchu in equal amounts is equally effective. Add horsetail if urinary incontinence is a feature.

Diet

To flush out the bladder, drink 250 ml of water every hour until symptoms improve. It is better if this is barley water, as it soothes the urinary tract. If you do not like the taste, flavour it with ginger or a herbal tea. One cup of barley is simmered in nine cups of water for thirty minutes. Add some lemon peel and allow the liquid to cool. Drink this several times daily. Slippery elm is also very soothing to the urinary tract: make 1 teaspoon into a gruel and then add as much water as you wish. Flavour this, as the taste is not very exciting. You may add one teaspoon of buchu leaves to either the barley or slippery elm drink, as this has the same anti-bacterial effect as golden seal. Take this four times daily.

Alkalise the tissues with fruit and vegetable juices (especially watermelon), salads and fruit. Eat pumpkin and watermelon seeds.

Supplements

- **Vitamin C** - 500 mg hourly as calcium ascorbate until symptoms improve and then reduce the frequency of dosage.
- **Vitamin A** - 25,000 IU daily or beta carotene 45 mg daily.
- **Zinc** - 50 mg daily.
- **Garlic** - 1 g three times daily.
- **Tissue salts kali chlor., ferrum phos.** and **natrum phos.** - two hourly.

Herbs

- **Golden seal, mountain grape** or **barberry** - 1 g three times daily.
- **Uva ursi** - 1 g three times daily.

The above herbs are specific to staphylococcus and E. coli and will clear infection in a few days. They work best in slightly alkaline urine. Marshmallow herb alkalises. A good blend of herbs for urinary infection is as follows:

Uva ursi, buchu, fennel, golden seal, dandelion and **marshmallow.**

Make this up as a tincture in equal amounts and take one teaspoon four times daily or blend the dry herbs together and make a tea with 30 g (1 oz) and half a litre of water and drink one third three times daily. The tea will have a bitter taste. Health food stores sell herbs in capsule form and you will be able to find a blend similar to this one. If there is no dandelion in it, buy this as a dried herb and make a tea to go with your herbal capsules. Cornsilk or golden rod herbs are also useful and palatable in tea form.

Homeopathy

Take 30C hourly if necessary for a few doses and then three times daily until the condition subsides. Match the symptoms correctly or there will be no improvement in the condition.

- **Cantharis** - for frequent strong urging before, during and after passing urine. Severe cutting or stabbing pain during urination. Frantic with pain, better for rubbing. This is the most commonly required remedy.
- **Sarsaparilla** - for stinging, cutting pain in the urethra only at the end of passing urine.
- **Mercurius** - fits all the classic symptoms. Pain is severe any time but worse at night and when not urinating. Person may have bad breath and sour perspiration.
- **Berberis** - for a frequent desire to urinate. The pain occurs during and after urinating and moves from the bladder to the urethra or from the urethra to the thighs and back. Worse for movement or jarring. The urethra burns even more when not urinating.
- **Pulsatilla** - for the gentle, weepy type with smarting and burning that is not severe, but more chronic. Worse lying on the back.
- **Aconite** - profuse urination, burning in the urethra, anxiety at the beginning of the flow. Worse in the evening, night and in a warm room.
- **Thuja** - for a urethra which is swollen and inflamed. Frequency and pain - urinary flow is split and small and there is a sensation of trickling afterwards. Desire is sudden, urgent and cannot be controlled. Worse at night from bed heat, cold damp air, after breakfast or from eating fat.
- **Apis** - for sharp stinging pain with swelling. Urine is scanty and hot. Worse for heat.
- **Staphysagria** - for a constant burning pain which starts after intercourse.

- **Tarentula** - for high fever, agonising pain and swollen bladder.

Prevention

This depends on the cause. If you are suffering from chronic cystitis due to high stress levels the only solution is to deal with the emotions. If the condition is caused by acidity in the body then the diet has to be altered so that it is 75% alkaline forming. This means loads of fruit or vegetables at every meal which can be reduced proportionally if you are eating soya beans, fresh coconut, buckwheat or millet. A deficiency of vitamin B6 can increase your susceptibility to urinary infections. Where cystitis is due to persistent infection, the following supplements will prevent the bacteria from adhering to the walls of the bladder:

- **Glucosamine as nag** - 500 mg 2 to 3 times daily
- **Cranberry concentrate** - 300 mg in capsule form or one half to one cup of unsweetened juice daily. **Blueberry juice** contains the same inhibitors as cranberry. This is not to cure an existing condition, but it is a very good preventative method.

Avoid chlorinated water, bubble baths and nylon underwear. Do not hold urine for long periods either. Drink enough water every day to pass clear urine all day long. Pay particular attention to washing hands and genitals before and after intercourse. Clean from front to back after a bowel movement. Wash in a bidet after passing urine.

12. Acne

Acne is the most common skin problem. It predominantly affects teenagers and involves an interaction between androgenic hormones, the skin and its normal bacteria. The problem is that the pores of the skin become blocked and skin bacteria then cause an inflammatory reaction with the resulting papules and pustules.

Acne patients show an increased conversion of the hormone testosterone to its more potent form and for this reason treatment is partly aimed at reducing the enzyme responsible by raising the intake of protein and reducing fat and carbohydrate in the diet.

When acne occurs in twenty to thirty-year olds, allergy normally plays a part. Even in teenagers, removing their particular food allergens can play a role in the reduction of lesions. Sometimes a deficient thyroid function is implicated or a general imbalance of female hormones. Poor skin care such as over washing and using cold tar soaps can aggravate acne.

Unbalanced diets with high levels of refined carbohydrate, high fat and low protein, increase acne. Unfortunately, this is the type of diet that many young people live on. Low fat sources of protein need to be increased and the carbohydrate must be of the whole variety, meaning that it must be unprocessed. Sugar and foods made from white flour such as bread, cakes, biscuits, pancakes, crumpet, pizza, pasta and bagels will increase the skins cholesterol levels and so the risk of blocked pores.

Teenagers so often eat high levels of refined flour that their sugar insulin interaction becomes unbalanced in the skin, and this may also trigger the inflammatory cascade. Certainly sugar suppresses the immune system's ability to fight infection. Removing these foods from the diet and adding glucose tolerance factor in the form of Brewer's yeast leads to a marked improvement on its own, which demonstrates the sugar intolerance factor. Studies indicate acne sufferers exhibit a skin intolerance to glucose, but not a blood intolerance. This is significantly improved by Brewer's yeast which contains chromium. As well as the refined carbohydrate, acne sufferers usually eat a lot of fat in the form of burgers, sausages, milk, cheese in white bread sandwiches and on toast and pizzas. The combination almost guarantees acne, especially as these foods crowd out the eating of fruit, vegetables, wholegrains, pulses and fish with all their important nutrients.

Treatment

Correct the diet.
Check on any hormone imbalances with blood or saliva tests.
Improve glucose tolerance.
Inhibit the enzyme which converts testosterone (5-alpha-reductase) with dietary control.
Improve the function of liver, bowel and kidneys to clear all toxins.
Replace nutrient deficiencies.
Check out food allergies

Diet

This should be largely alkaline forming, which means fruit and vegetables form a major part of the diet.
A large plate of vegetables at lunch and dinner and one should be totally raw. Include fresh garlic - nature's antibiotic.
Fruit at breakfast and in between meals.
Fish, and especially the oily type, at least three times weekly.
Eggs three times weekly provide excellent quality protein.
Organic or genuine wild meat is permitted if it is low in fat.
Low fat cottage cheese twice weekly in small servings.
Dried peas, beans, lentils and soya products like tofu for protein on the days that fish is not eaten.
Eat one or two servings daily of the following to make complete protein with the pulses and also provide quality carbohydrate: whole grains such as brown rice, millet, cornmeal, buckwheat, oats, barley, rye and wheat (wholewheat bread, pasta, pizza crust).
Sprouted seeds and pulses for meganutrients.

Raw nuts and seeds for essential polyunsaturated oils - sunflower, sesame, pumpkin and flaxseeds, almonds and walnuts.

A parsley and lemon juice drink half an hour before breakfast, with added barley greens or wheatgrass juice.

Herbal tea - especially fennel, peppermint and sarsaparilla.

Mineral water - six to eight glasses daily.

Brewers yeast - one teaspoon or six tablets twice daily.

Extra virgin olive oil is the only permitted oil for cooking and dressings.

One tablespoon of flaxseeds daily with warm water to improve bowel function.

Reduce

Meat, eggs, butter and cheese because of the fat and arachadonic acid content which leads to inflammatory chemicals. Farmed meat contains hormones which should be avoided; lamb is normally free of these, but has a very high fat content. Also reduce salt.

Avoid

All processed and refined foods. This means nearly all canned, packet and frozen foods, sugar, white flour, cornstarch, white rice and everything made from them. It also means no processed cereals; only natural sugar-free muesli or porridge grains.

Roasted and fried foods.

All animal fat, processed oils, margarines and all foods canned in oil (remove it from sardines and mackerel).

Tea, coffee, alcohol, chocolate, soft drinks, cordials and unfiltered tap water.

Foods to which you are allergic.

Dried fruit and concentrated fruit juice because the levels of fruit sugar are unnaturally high.

Milk as it increases the progesterone hormone in the blood.

Vitamin B12 supplements and inorganic iron as they aggravates acne.

The contraceptive pill as it reduces many essential vitamins and minerals.

Juices

Wheat or barley juice.

Lemon, grapefruit, beetroot (redbeet), and greens freshly pressed all improve liver function.

This diet is high in protein from pulses, grains and vegetables as well as animal sources, low in fat and contains quality complex carbohydrate. This pattern ensures the inhibition of the enzyme which converts testosterone. With low fat levels, free radicals are less likely to be generated and this is very important.

Treatment which encourages the production of antioxidants has been shown to improve acne markedly. Antioxidants mop up free radicals before they can do any harm. The low saturated fat content plus increased levels of oils from fish, nuts and seeds ensures inflammatory reactions are controlled and the anti-inflammatory prostaglandins E_1 and E_3 predominate. The inclusion of complex carbohydrate and the total avoidance of the refined type ensures that no glucose intolerance occurs in the skin.

Supplements of value

The supplements which follow are to prevent the blockage of the skin pores with sebum, provide a substitute for antibiotics, mop up inflammatory chemicals and provide antioxidant cover. If your acne is caused by an imbalance of oestrogen and progesterone premenstrually, add magnesium 200 mg twice daily to the following.

- **Vitamin A** - 100,000 IU daily for three months is safe but more effective if given with the other antioxidants. Do not take this if you might become pregnant.
- **Vitamin E** - 400 IU once or twice daily.
- **Vitamin C** - 500 mg three times daily.
- **Selenium** - 200 mcg daily.

- **Zinc** - 50 mg once or twice daily as citrate or as effervescent zinc sulphate.
- **B complex** - 25 mg daily with folic acid at 5 mg and no B12. Folic acid has proven beneficial in its own right.
- **Vitamin B6** - 50 mg twice daily if acne flairs premenstrually.
- **Vitamin B5 (pantothenic acid)** - reduces sebum production. A study involving one hundred Chinese under thirty years old, used 10 g daily to great effect, but it is possible that much lower doses may be just as useful.
- **Chromium** - 400 mcg daily as polynicotinate if you cannot take the Brewer's yeast.
- **GLA as evening primrose oil** - 500 mg twice daily or half the dose of **borage oil**.
- **Flaxseed oil** - 3,000 mg daily if not eating oily fish.
- **Tissue salts - ferrum phos** and **kali chlor.** - inhibits the formation of the red sore papules.
- **Silica** - clears the pus.
- **Benzoyl peroxide 5% gel** - topically applied at night after washing.

Inclusion of the first six ingredients is particularly important as well as following the diet. Others are all very useful and worth considering and a period of blood, liver and lymph cleansing with herbs would also be of great value.

Zinc - is very important for all skin conditions as it is involved in healing, immune system activity and maintaining serum levels of vitamin A. The levels need to be high as low dosage increases testosterone conversion which in turn increases acne. Studies have also noted that high levels of zinc are as effective as the tetracyclines which are used long term by the medical profession. However twelve weeks of supplementation is necessary before results become apparent. People with acne are usually deficient in zinc when compared with those who are free of this problem.

Vitamin E regulates the blood levels of activated vitamin A and has an important regulating effect on female hormones. It requires its partner, selenium, in order to function properly.

Vitamin A prevents the blockage of the pores with sebum but the dose needs to be very high. One study found that this vitamin was only effective at 300,000 IU daily, but in my experience lower doses are fine if the other antioxidants are taken at the same time.

If the dose of vitamin A is too high, dry skin and chapped lips will develop, followed by headaches, fatigue, muscle and joint pains. However, this is rare even at higher doses than 100,000 IU daily over three months. Stopping treatment will immediately reverse toxicity.

Herbs

These are for blood, lymph and liver cleansing.

- **Echinacea** - 2 g daily or 500 mg of extract.
- **Marigold** - 1 g daily or 250 mg of extract.
- **Dandelion root** - 2 g three times daily.

A good blend is: **Dandelion root, echinacea, burdock, red clover, poke root and golden seal.** Mix equal amounts of tincture and take one teaspoon twice daily. There are many blends on the market in capsule form so ask in your local health food store for a good blood and lymph cleansing blend of herbs.

Homeopathy

Dose 6C twice daily.

- **Sulphur** - for long-standing obstinate cases with rough hard skin that is made worse by washing. The teenager is untidy with jumbled clothes drawers and leaves the bathroom in a mess.
- **Kali brom.** - chronic conditions, itchy spots, restless sleep and unpleasant dreams.
- **Hepar sulph.** - for large pustules.
- **Pulsatilla** - for acne in pale blondes who are sensitive and weepy. The condition is made worse by rich food.

- **Ant. tart.** - for obstinate cases with more pustules than red spots.
- **Calc. sulph.** - for the blind pimples and also for yellow discharge or crusts. Acne does not heal quickly.
- **Silicea** - for acne which scars easily.
- **Myristica** - brings large spots to a head and clears them more quickly than hepar sulph.

Others

Daily exercise and sunshine.
Dry skin brushing and hot and cold showers daily to improve lymph and blood circulation.
Wash with calendula soap for its healing effect. Cornstarch washes have an anti-inflammatory effect.
Improve thyroid function if necessary.
Colon cleanse if necessary.
Cold pressed aloe vera gel can be applied to the face.
Tea tree oil dabbed on spots neat three times daily or use it in water as a wash. This essential oil is a powerful antiseptic.
Bran face packs help. Add half a teaspoon of baking powder to half a cup of bran. Soak it fifteen minutes and apply to the face for the same length of time. Rinse off with a cider vinegar solution of one part to eight parts water.
Propolis tincture may be applied to the skin. This is another natural antibiotic like garlic.

13. Weight Loss

There is an optimal level of body fat for everyone and once that is exceeded, the system feels sluggish and uncomfortable, with reduced energy levels. Very few people who are prone to gaining pounds are able to consistently maintain their normal weight, resulting in frequent bouts of dieting and a steady increase in fat levels over the decades.

It has been scientifically proven time and time again that dieting slows metabolism, so each time a diet is embarked upon the rate of energy production is slowed down a little more. Eventually very few calories are needed to sustain life. Missing meals slows the metabolism. At 1200 calories (5000 kilojoules) a day the metabolic rate also slows; at 800 calories (2400 kilojoules), the body's thermo-regulation by the hypothalamus in the brain is damaged, reducing the rate further. However, a reduced metabolism caused by dieting does not affect the fat cells which are used for storing waste from junk food. The body simply burns protein instead of fat for energy. Rebound eating then puts fat into muscle cells which become flabby. A major source of dangerous chemicals are 'diet' soft drinks.

The very process of weighing, measuring and consulting a calorie counter encourages a dieting mentality which implies that this eating pattern is temporary. The mind of the dieter sees a return to another eating habit which is viewed as normal. The only successful way of maintaining an ideal weight is to eat in the same manner at all times, reducing solid food a little when a few pounds have crept up. Exercise and a positive outlook on life are of prime importance, as is self-esteem. If you do not like yourself, weight increase is more likely. Emotional problems upset the nervous and hormonal control over weight.

Metabolism

There are a great many reasons for weight gain and eating the wrong type of food is one. Some also have a genetic tendency to store food because of slow metabolism and this has to be speeded up with regular exercise and supplements. A poor digestive function will slow metabolism, so reasons for this must be examined if necessary. There may be a deficiency of gastric acid and enzymes which means that food is not broken down properly and therefore not digested adequately. The end result is a lack of nutrients and the formation of toxins in the bowel which then get re-absorbed into the blood and tissues. Sometimes enzymes are not formed because the diet lacks the necessary nutrients over a prolonged period.

Where the thyroid function is slightly below par it is known as sub-clinical hypothyroidism, which also leads to a slow metabolic rate. However, this condition will not show in a blood test. Rather, it is necessary to look for symptoms of the condition such as low basal body temperature, low gastric acid secretion and indigestion, fluid retention, vague depression, dry horny callused skin on the feet, falling hair, a tendency to constipation, raised cholesterol, heart irregularities, or poor wound healing. Where hypothyroidism exists, it has hitherto been felt advisable to avoid foods which inhibits the thyroid's uptake of iodine. These foods are white cabbage, collards, red cabbage, brussel sprouts, cauliflower, broccoli, pakchoi, cress, swede, turnip, kale, soya beans, ground nuts and mustard seeds. However, recent research indicates that a daily supplement of iodine overrides the problem so that these very beneficial foods can be eaten without fear of goitre or hypothyroidism developing.

There are many possible reasons for a slow thyroid, but a major cause is unbalanced female hormones. High levels of oestrogen will suppress the output of the thyroid hormone so if you suffer PMS as well as a weight problem, your extra kilograms could all be due to an oestrogen-progesterone imbalance.

Food allergies are another reason for ever-increasing weight and fluid retention. In this situation, it is a great joy to discover that abstention from a single food group removes the battle of the bulge. If the allergic reaction occurs in the pancreas, it can affect the output of digestive enzymes as well as blood sugar control. Those who do not exercise are telling their bodies that fat-burning enzymes are not required. These enzymes are stored in the muscle energy centres (mitochondria) and if a person exercises, muscle makes more mitochondria to produce more energy by burning increased amounts of fat.

Brown fat

This type of fat is a rich source of energy which is rapidly converted for use in the body. It is full of mitochondria with their fat-burning enzymes. Brown fat is activated by the thyroid and adrenal glands, aerobic exercise, caffeine and a low fat diet. Essential polyunsaturated fats from oily fish and evening primrose oil also increase brown fat. Diets high in protein and fat, poison brown fat whereas high complex carbohydrate (whole grains, pulses) and low fat diets activate it. One study showed that Vitamin C along with evening primrose oil increased brown fat within three to four weeks, however, large doses were needed and 8 g of evening primrose oil were shown to be more effective than 4 g.

Set point

Research has found that everyone has a programmed 'set point' or 'fat point'. This means that whatever fat cells are present, the body keeps them full so that if a cell loses some fat a message goes to the brain to tell the individual to eat more. This is one reason for the overpowering desire to indulge which causes dieting to fail and a rebound weight gain to occur. It is nothing to do with willpower. Obese people have more and larger fat cells and the set point keeps them full. Every time dieting and rebound eating occurs, the fat point is set higher in order to protect the body against future bouts of starvation. The only way to halt to this process is to *stop going on diets.*

Set point levels seem to be related to insulin sensitivity. It has been found that if the set point is high (as in overweight people), the fat cells do not respond to insulin and therefore will not release fat for fuel. Conversely, insulin will stimulate the production of new fat cells in those who consume excessive sugar and white flour so that these foods can be converted to fat for storage. In order to lower the programmed set point we must avoid foods which stimulate insulin outpourings (see "glycaemic foods" below), eat a healthy raw food diet and exercise. Once the set point is down, fat cells will shrink.

Slimmed down, fat people initially have an enhanced ability to produce and store fat because the fat cells are still large. Therefore if food intake is increased, those cells will fill very quickly. Fat cell production works on the ratchet effect whereby cells increase in numbers rapidly, but it is impossible to turn back and reduce the actual number. They can only be shrunken and this process involves a long period of never overeating once the weight has been reduced.

Glycaemic foods

Foods which stimulate excessive insulin production out of proportion to their calorie content are termed 'glycaemic foods'. They maintain or aggravate obesity and should be avoided by anyone wishing to lose weight. Insulin is rapidly activated by white flour and sugary snacks, whereas a nut/raisin/oatmeal snack has 70% less effect on insulin secretion. Generally speaking, the high fibre foods have a low glycaemic effect, but not always. As an example, a banana is highly glycaemic in spite of containing high fibre levels. Foods have been given glycaemic ratings beginning with glucose at 100. White bread, maltose and honey are almost as close with a rating of 95. Even wheat cereal and whole wheat bread score between 75 and 85 with wheat pasta at 60 to 65. Starchy vegetables like potatoes, carrots, corn and parsnips are also relatively high but the glycaemic effect is reduced when eaten with green leafy vegetables and some protein. Rice, other whole grains, comes in at a moderate 50 and the really high fibred dried peas, beans and lentils are at a low 20 to 30. Most green vegetables and whole fruits are also very low. Surprisingly, fruit sugar (fructose) also has a low glycaemic rating.

Every time a high glycaemic food is eaten, an outpouring of insulin occurs, preventing fat cells from shedding fat as the insulin converts sugar into fat instead of energy. Chocolate cake followed by a missed meal to make up for the sin, may have a calorie balancing effect, but will have the undesired result of maintaining fat cell insensitivity to insulin. This means that fat cells will not shed fat for energy when the insulin attaches to them. Furthermore, when insulin is released, it clears sugar from the blood into fat storage depots, leaving a hypoglycaemic effect (low blood sugar), which in turn leads to increased hunger pangs. Complex carbohydrate from green vegetables, most fruits and non-wheat whole grain does not trigger insulin and therefore does not trigger sweet cravings.

The slimming organisation, Weight Watchers, aside from weighing and measuring all foods, allows canned foods, white bread and crispbread, all of which are highly glycaemic. No wonder so many people who join this well-meaning group need life membership! I have observed many women trying to lose weight by moderate eating instead of dieting as such, who tend towards highly glycaemic foods, for instance, toast and a banana for breakfast followed by a sandwich for lunch and a small pasta dinner. The calories are low but fat burning is not possible because insulin is being triggered at every meal.

In order to beat those cravings for sweet food and to avoid outpourings of insulin, a diet which avoids glycaemic carbohydrates and stimulants is very important. This means eating lots of green vegetables along with pulses and unprocessed grains - but no wheat in any form. Pay attention to your blood type here when choosing the proportion of whole grains and pulses, as this could also make the difference between losing and gaining weight.

The control of blood sugar levels depends on chromium as well as avoiding glycaemic foods. Levels of this trace mineral reduce as we grow older so supplementation is often necessary. Many other nutrients are also necessary to ensure that sugars are converted to energy rather than fat: vitamins C and B complex, zinc and magnesium.These are also essential to hormone balance and therefore proper thyroid function.

Biochemical individuality

In order to maintain proper weight levels it is important to give the body the type of fuel on which it runs best. We are all biochemically different so note which foods suit you best. My book "You Don't Have To Feel Unwell" goes into great detail in this field so I will focus only on the blood groups[1] here. In my clinical experience, it is true that eating according to body type, reduces weight, even if this involves more calories than normally taken while trying to lose weight slowly.

Treatment

Alter the diet to reset the fat point to provide a lifelong eating pattern.

Exercise.

Treat malfunctions such as hypothyroidism or low stomach acid.

Determine whether food allergies are present.

Diet

This should be high in fibre and complex carbohydrate as well as being alkaline producing. Eat a wide variety of fruits, vegetables and sprouted products as well as nuts, permitted grains and all types of pulses. In order to lose weight 75% of food should be raw.

Fruit and vegetables must form 50% of the diet. Ideally a large plate of vegetables is eaten twice daily with all other food treated as a side dish. Eat fruit for breakfast and between meals only. Drink a glass of juiced vegetables daily and sprinkle some seaweed on salads for its high mineral content. Fruits and vegetables detoxify the tissues remove waste and increase

1 See page 187

metabolism. If you do not eat sprouted food, fruit and vegetables should form 75% of your diet.

Sprouted food should form 25% of the diet for top-rated health and energy levels. Buy a book which teaches you how to sprout nuts, seeds, beans and lentils. They regenerate enzymes, hormones and cells and the vitamin/mineral level of a food is increased by 200 to 2000% by being sprouted.

The following foods should form 25% of the diet and be treated as side dishes. Choose according to your blood group (at end of chapter) and see how that suits you before doing any fine tuning.

Whole grains, particularly millet, brown rice and quinoa. Restrict oats, barley and rye to once daily.

Nuts and seeds, unroasted and unsalted. These are vital for their essential polyunsaturated oils.

Low fat dairy foods in small amounts.

Fish, chicken, eggs.

Soya beans, lentils and other dried peas and beans.

Extra virgin olive oil for dressings.

Brewer's yeast and sardines depress the appetite centre.

Include chromium rich herbs and foods on a daily basis: Brewers yeast, egg yolk, whole grains, mushrooms, lettuce, tomatoes, beans, onions, liver, clams, cheese, caraway, coriander, mace, cinnamon, nutmeg, poppy seeds, cumin, cloves and bayleaves.

Avoid

All processed and refined food because the additives have to be stored in fat cells.

Glycaemic foods - sugar; wheat (bread, pasta crackers, etc); cornstarch and everything made from them; all processed grains and flours; bananas, sweet grapes, fruit juices and honey.

Alcohol, cigarettes and coffee as they are stimulants which release sugar stores and unbalance blood sugar levels.

Avoid the above foods for a period, even after weight has been lost, in order to shrink the fat cells.

Fats from dairy products, meats, mayonnaise and processed oils.

Coffee, squashes and carbonated drinks, including diet drinks and sweeteners which are full of chemicals needing storage in fat cells.

Excessive protein as it is void of fibre and creates acidity in the tissues.

Snacks; as studies indicate, overweight people eat bigger meals after snacks than if nothing is eaten between meals. Individuals of normal weight decrease the food intake following a snack.

Foods causing allergies as the hypothalamus, which regulates the appetite, has a histamine receptor. The histamine from allergic reactions prevents the appetite centre from being turned off.

Counting calories because it develops a dieting mentality.

Constipation as eliminated chemicals are reabsorbed.

Restrict

Foods which do not fit your blood group.

Dairy foods to a little low fat cottage cheese, live yoghurt or a scraping of butter.

Starchy vegetables to small servings in favour of more greens.

Meat to moderate servings three times weekly. Use fish on the other days unless you are a natural vegetarian. Restrict salt.

General

Eat slowly and chew well. A high fibre diet ensures excretion of fat, better digestive enzyme production and increased glucose tolerance. It induces a feeling of fullness after moderate caloric intake.

Eat three meals a day and do not eat late at night.

Follow food combining rules. (see “You Don’t Have To Feel Unwell” for detailed information). Basically this means do not combine protein and starch at the same meal. Eat only as much as you need.

Some Menu Ideas

Breakfast

Fresh fruit, live plain yoghurt and a few chopped fresh nuts - no bananas or fruit juice.

One or two eggs.

Rye bread or oatmeal occasionally.

Millet, brown rice, quinoa or amaranth porridge with a little skimmed milk and a little fructose if necessary.

Lunch

A large raw salad with sprouted foods in significant amounts.

A side dish of one of the following; low fat cottage cheese, brown rice salad, buckwheat (a seed), quinoa, or millet pasta, tofu or pulses made into a salad with yoghurt dressing and fresh herbs.

Home-made soup for warm food in the winter.

Dinner

A large plate of vegetables and sprouted foods, stir-fried (grease-free), steamed or raw, or a mixture of both raw and cooked.

A side dish of fish, chicken, lamb fillet, egg or vegetarian protein as at lunch.

Drinks

Herbal tea, mineral water, miso, vegetable juices and broths. Diluted fruit juices may be added occasionally once your ideal weight is reached.

Dressings

Extra virgin olive oil and cider vinegar with garlic, herbs and French mustard.

Yoghurt and flavourings like horseradish or tahini, lemon and soya sauce or mint, garlic and cucumber. You could also make a tomato based sauce with herbs or spices.

The more raw food you include in the diet, the less food you will want and the higher your metabolic rate. Toxins will be destroyed and the fat point reset. The way to permanent weight loss is through exercise and a diet which is high in fibre (from fruit vegetables and complex carbohydrate), moderate in protein and low in fat.

Supplements of value

Adult doses

- **GLA as evening primrose oil** - 4,000 mg daily, or **borage oil,** 2,000 mg. To help break down fat stores if you are more than 10% overweight.
- **Carnitine** - 250 mg of this amino acid three times daily with water half an hour before food to increase fat burning inside cells.
- **Tyrosine** - 500 mg of this amino acid once or twice daily with water, half an hour before food for thyroid hormone production and a feeling of well-being.
- **Zinc** - 25 mg daily for enzyme production, to activate thyroxine and control the appetite.
- **Potassium iodide** - 200 to 400 mcg daily for thyroxine production
- **Magnesium** - 200 to 400 mg daily.
- **B complex** - 50 mg daily for fat metabolism and blood sugar control.
- **Pancreatin** - 250 to 500 mg between meals helps to cut down food intake.
- **Flaxseed** - one tablespoon daily prevents constipation.
- **Chromium** - 100 mcg daily as glucose tolerance factor (GTF) or chromium polynicotinate if sugar craving is a problem.
- **Selenium** - 200 mcg daily is an essential part of an enzyme involved in thyroid function. This means that the metabo-

lism, and therefore the ability to lose weight, is damaged by a lack of this mineral.

- **Pantothenic acid** (vitamin B5) - a nutrition study reported in 1995 indicated an average weekly weight loss of 1 to 2 kg in one hundred overweight people. They were given 2.5 g of this vitamin four times daily. It is thought that fat burning was speeded up by this nutrient.

Herbs

- **Dandelion** - 4 g daily or as a tea for a liver cleanse and to assist the liver in detoxification.
- **Germander** - as a tea between meals. It suppresses the appetite and weight gain but does not have an amphetamine action.
- **Tamarind plant** (Garcinia cambogia) - contains an acid (HCA) which inhibits the enzyme responsible for converting excess glucose to fat instead of glycogen (stored sugar waiting to be used for energy). This acid will also increase the rate of fat burning and reduce the synthesis of cholesterol. Many exciting studies have proven the benefit of this plant which is most effective when given with chromium.

Exercise

This must be aerobic to increase the body's oxygen supply, to increase efficient fat discarding and to raise fat-burning enzymes. If oxygen levels are low, the system feels sluggish and there is a strong desire to eat the wrong food. This always happens in individuals who are mentally or physically low. Fat stores increase, muscle and bone density is lost and skin thins and wrinkles when oxygen is depleted. Deep breathing exercises are also important for increasing the oxygenation of the body.

Exercise is an important feature in lowering the set point, eliminating toxins, improving sluggish liver function and especially for increasing metabolism. The ideal form of exercise is sustained and at 60% of maximum only. It has been found that weight loss is higher if exercise is not at 80% of maximum. This is because where exercise is too intense, the muscles cannot take in enough oxygen. Rebounding on a mini-trampoline is of value, as is brisk walking, gentle jogging or dancing, swimming, rowing or skating. Stop and start sports like tennis are not aerobic. To ascertain your safe aerobic rate for weight loss, use the following equation: 220, minus age times 0.6 or 0.8.

Meditation and visualisation

These techniques can be successfully used to help you lose weight. Use these periods to instruct yourself not to eat between meals or constantly raid the refrigerator. Use visualisation to see the fat self shrinking into just the sort of shape you require and then see yourself remaining this way permanently. The mind is all powerful so make it work for you.

Blood group diets

This eating pattern is not set in stone but is a good starting point. Any food to which you are allergic in a particular blood group, should be eliminated until it is safe to eat it again. Unsuitable products should be treated like occasional treats - never part of the daily routine

O Group diet

Unsuitable fuel

Fatty meats like beef, lamb and pork and chicken leg and wing. Dairy products - milk, cheese, butter and yoghurt except for unpasteurised milk products which are low in fat and taken in moderation 2 to 3 times weekly.

Wheat bread and wheat pasta as well as cereal grains, and reduce other grains to once daily. Some can tolerate an oatmeal cereal for breakfast and soya bread is classed as good fuel.

Good fuel

Fruit and vegetables of all types in abundance.

Fish and low fat meat: liver, kidney, organic beef, lamb fillet, chicken breast and wild venison. Eat these once daily only.

Eggs in moderation - 4 to 5 weekly.

Pulses - chickpeas, soya beans, tofu, black-eyed peas, red kidney beans, green and red beans, lentils - including soya bread.

Low fat nuts and seeds, such as sunflower and pumpkin seeds and almonds.

Small servings occasionally of brown rice and cornmeal, but only once daily.

Starch is better found in starchy vegetables - potato, pumpkin, parsnip, yam and carrot.

Pasta made of buckwheat or quinoa, which are seeds and not grains. These can also be bought in grain-like form for cooking as a substitute for rice.

O group people have a requirement for high protein diets and cannot be vegetarian, but equally the diet needs to be low in fat. The pulses are an excellent source of protein and can replace animal protein on some days in the week.

The O blood group is the original one dating back before the ice age. These people ate small amounts which did not include farmed grains or dairy products. Their meat source was fish from the sea and wild meat which is very low in saturated fat.

A Group diet

Unsuitable fuel

Pulses - dried beans, peas, lentils and peanuts (except soya as tofu, soya milk and miso).

Meat of any type.

Wheat. Some can tolerate it 1 to 2 times weekly.

Dairy products, although some are well adapted to low fat varieties 2 to 3 times weekly.

Good fuel

Vegetables of all types and in abundance, but use avocado sparingly.

Beans, when sprouted and used in salad, e.g. alfalfa, mung and soya.

Fruit in moderation.

All grains (except wheat) but use only whole grains, e.g. brown rice, oats, barley, rye, millet, cornmeal and pasta made of these grains.

Polyunsaturated nuts and seeds - unsalted and unroasted.

All types of fish but only 2 to 3 times weekly.

Eggs 2 to 3 weekly but only boiled or poached.

An A group person is a natural vegetarian and protein is derived from whole grains plus soya products if they do not eat fish.

B Group diet

Unsuitable fuel

Chicken.

Good fuel

Meat (except chicken) and fish but in small servings. Macrobiotics are suitable with dairy products added in the fermented state only.

Vegetables in good servings twice daily and fruit in moderation.

Fermented dairy products such as yoghurt, quark and unpasteurised cheeses like brie and camembert.

Eggs 3 to 4 times weekly.

Grains in abundance but eat as whole grains for good health, e.g. brown rice, millet wholewheat bread and pasta instead of the white nutritionally deficient type.
Nuts and seeds, especially sesame seed paste (tahini).
Pulses of all kinds, but in moderation.

AB group diet

Unsuitable fuel

Meat of any type and wheat products.

Good fuel

Vegetarian is most suitable.
Fermented unpasteurised dairy products such as yoghurt, quark and camembert type cheeses.
Vegetables of all types and in abundance, but use avocado sparingly.
Fruit in moderation.
All grains (except wheat), but use only whole grain, e.g. brown rice, oats, barley, rye, millet, cornmeal and pasta made of these grains.
Pulses of all types, including soya bread.
Eggs 3 to 4 times weekly.
Polyunsaturated nuts and seeds - unsalted and unroasted.
All types of fish, but only 2 to 3 times weekly.
These people do very well on abundant diets. They are well suited to vegetarianism and the only ones completely adapted to the nightshade family of foods - potatoes, tomatoes, capsicum peppers, aubergines and tamarillos.

PART 3 - PREGNANCY

Pregnancy

Women of this modern age are becoming increasingly aware of the importance of being completely tuned into their unborn child from a very early stage in the pregnancy. Being one with your child is as important during pregnancy as after the infant is born. For this reason it is a great shame to be so caught up in a career or other activities that there is little time to be with your child on a mental level except when you sit down at night. Pregnancy is a time to feel special and be in tune with nature. Your unborn child will pick up the positive vibrations generated by a mother who is enjoying her pregnancy. It is so important to decide to become pregnant only when you have already made time for a newcomer in your life and not think of the pregnancy as nine months breathing space to continue in a busy life as though not much has changed.

I think every women should experience a rebirthing session before becoming pregnant, because it is a real eye-opener in terms of how a baby feels during the birthing process. This method taps into the subconscious to understand your feelings while in the womb and during the birthing process. Until you have consciously experienced the emotions surrounding your own birth, it is difficult to truly understand the loneliness and fears that an infant may experience during birth. I have talked to many women who have under gone this as therapy and their own birth experiences covered a wide range of emotions. Some feared being unable to get out of the birth canal, others did not want to leave what they perceived as a safe warm environment and a few panicked half way and wanted to go back inside. Many were aware of the fact that they were emotionally cut off from their mother at the most crucial time in the whole nine months and felt devastated and very fearful. This is why it is so important to build a loving relationship with your unborn child from the beginning. It is especially crucial to not split off into your own pain just as your baby has its greatest need for mother's love, encouragement and support.

Long before your delivery time is due, make sure that the environment will be just as you wish. Once an infant is born it is capable of registering fear at being carried away from mother just when it most needs to be cuddled by her. The noise, bright lights and general hustle and bustle of a hospital birthing room are alarming. Soft music should be played in the room and do choose something that you know your child enjoys - this will give it confidence. As soon as possible after delivery, the baby should be allowed to lie on the mother's chest where it can feel the familiar heartbeat and come to terms with the new, strange, big world it has entered.

Throughout the pregnancy, your child needs to feel loved by both parents, so remember that it will be tuned into father as well as mother and both must talk to it every day. It will not understand if father is not around for long periods. It has been established that a child's experience in the womb has a great deal to do with the mother's personality and behaviour patterns in life. A mother who is calm and delighting in her pregnancy is much more likely to produce a contented, smiling child. If there is dissension, tension or unhappiness in the family, the unborn child will feel it. When mother pumps out stress hormones like adrenalin, they go straight through the placenta and affect the child. It may react immediately by kicking or moving about as though distressed. Statistics show that children born of stressed women are more likely to have colic and cry a lot. Their birth weights are often low and later they are more likely than other children to be hyperactive.

Convert any negative thoughts into positive ones as they arise and make your baby part of your life from the beginning. Talk to it throughout the day as if it were an adult because the little soul inside does have the wisdom of ages. Sing to it and play soft music. As you near the fourth month, your child becomes very sensitive to all sounds and by the seventh month will communicate a preference for a certain type of music. You will be able to sense this by its movements. Most babies enjoy Vivaldi and Bach, but they can also develop a liking for certain popular songs. This belief is proven by mothers who notice that their young ones will stop playing and listen intently to a piece of music which they enjoyed in the womb. I know a mother whose unborn child clearly enjoyed Bach, but was quite definite about its dislike of Pavarotti.

As you talk to your baby, do not forget to tell it that you love it. You may think that it is not necessary to state the obvious, but remember that none of us tires of being told that we are loved: your baby needs the constant reassurance. Touch is very important, so stroke the baby often and especially when you talk to it. In the later months it is possible to give your baby a daily massage from top to toe. Do it because it will love it. All of these sensations make your baby feel loved, wanted and completely tuned in to its parent.

This chapter is not intended to focus on the mundane as there are a great number of books written for pregnancy. I shall touch on the well known and concentrate on the more unusual.

Diet

Do not eat for two. If you focus on eating only what is healthy and eating only until you have had enough, all will be well. The PMS diet (Part 2, chapter 1) is a good general one and, unless you suffer low blood sugar, do not eat between meals. However if you are having a rough time with pregnancy sickness, you may find that it helps to eat little and often until this phase has passed. The protein allowance in your diet should be higher than normal but, rather than adding more animal foods, learn to use pulses and whole grains for their protein content. Extra protein is necessary to provide the building blocks for making a baby, but the protein from vegetable sources is just as good as that from animal as long as you eat both whole grains and pulses. Added benefits are that pulses add other nutrients which are not available in animal protein and the fat levels will be lowered. In fact pulses actually clear fats from the blood-stream to the liver and gall bladder, to be disposed of in the bowel.

All grains should be whole and not processed - experiment with using unusual grains like millet, quinoa, spelt, amaranth and buck-wheat. Some of these are not technically grains but are presented in grain form as cereals, pastas and flour. Change from pretty packaged cereals to porridge oats or unsweetened muesli and buy wholegrain breads and pastas. If you do not like wheat in this form, health food stores stock pastas made from buckwheat, corn, millet, spelt and quinoa. They taste wonderful. Shop regularly in your local health food store for a wide variety of interesting and healthy foods.

Eat a large serving of vegetables twice daily, ensuring that half is eaten raw as salad or juice for the living enzymes which are vital to health. Fruit should be eaten between every meal and it is a good habit to drink a freshly-made juice daily. For this you can use fruit, but a mixture of juiced vegetables is of greater benefit - canned varieties do nothing to increase your health as they contain no living enzymes.

Make sure that essential fatty acids in the form of unroasted, unsalted walnuts, flax, sunflower, sesame and pumpkin seeds, soya products and oily fish are a regular part of the diet, as these are vital to the health of your baby. Stay away from those processed polyunsaturated oils, shortenings and margarines found in the supermarkets. These are toxic to everyone's health and will block the activity of the essential natural polyunsaturates in foods. For cooking you should use extra virgin olive oil, a little coconut oil or butter. Natural foods are always better in terms of building health - just do not overdo the fats.

From the 25th week onwards, an ingredient of oily fish (DHA) is vital for the rapidly developing brain and immune system; the infant requires this after birth as well. It is not present in infant formulas and, in fact, infants who are not breastfed have been found to lose DHA for eight weeks after birth. These babies should have traces of fish oil added to their bottle feeds frequently throughout the day, as infant formulas do not contain DHA. The precursors of DHA (oils in seeds, walnuts and soya beans) have proven to be of little use as a source of this fatty acid in newborn infants, presumably because they are unable to convert them easily. In breast fed infants, DHA comes through the mother's diet, but in vegetarian women the level is reduced by at least half.

Where the mother's diet is deficient in omega 3 fatty acids (from oily fish, flax or pumpkin seeds) DHA is not formed in the infant in adequate amounts, which means that the immune and nervous systems will be poorly developed. The results could be the development of allergies such as eczema, asthma and colic, anxiety and other emotional disorders, as well as hyperactivity and learning disabilities. The incidence of all these conditions has exploded in the last two generations and this coincides with the rapidly increasing intake of toxic processed polyunsaturated oils used for cooking and present in almost all packaged foods as vegetable oil, margarine or shortening. These oils are damaged omega 6 fats, with the molecular structure of plastic. They interfere with the activity of natural polyunsaturated fats (in raw nuts and seeds and oily fish) in developing the brain, nervous and immune systems in the unborn child. If the mother continues on this path while breast-feeding it can lead to a lifetime of health problems for the child. Bottle fed infants receive formula with the same heat-damaged omega 6 oil which further exacerbates the lack of DHA.

For advice on calcium intake, see the chapter on osteoporosis for a list of calcium foods to eat in place of milk. As members of the human race, we were not designed to drink another animal's milk. Pasteurised dairy products cause many illnesses and are a major cause of food allergies in infants. These children become sensitised in the womb and once born can develop allergic problems like colic and poor sleeping habits. Take a calcium supplement during pregnancy rather than milk.

If varicose veins become a problem, strengthen the blood vessel walls with onion, garlic, buckwheat, oats and okra and the bioflavonoid, rutin. However the latter should be avoided in the first three months of pregnancy.

Macrobiotic diet

Macrobiotic mothers have been found to have decreasing amounts of zinc, calcium, magnesium, iron, vitamin B12 and saturated fat in their breast milk. This is because the high levels of phytates in their grains attache to the minerals in the bloodstream and removes them from the body. The only way to avoid this problem is to sprout, ferment or soak the grains for long periods before cooking or eating raw. A child deficient in B12 is irritable, apathetic, and refuses solid food. If not detected quickly, physical and intellectual development regresses and the infant fails to thrive. This will probably not become obvious until four to eight months of age.

Preventing allergy

If you or your husband have food allergies you are very likely to produce a child prone to allergy - it may even be sensitised to certain foods while still in the womb. For this reason it is important to avoid daily eating of common allergens: wheat, milk products, eggs, chicken, soya beans, citrus fruits, peanuts, sugar, food colourings, potatoes and tomatoes. All of these foods should be eaten on a rotation basis which means once every three to four days only, to lessen the risk of developing an allergy in the newborn infant. If that happens, life is rough for the mother because, not only does she have to avoid her own allergens, but as long as she is breast-feeding she has to also avoid her baby's allergens.

Allergic reactions can take many forms, of which rhinitis attacks are only one. Most recurring ailments in children are due to an allergic reaction to a common food. Some of the more usual problems associated with allergy are: colic, hard dry stools or diarrhoea, runny noses, ear infections, hyperactivity, poor concentration and learning difficulties, sleep disturbances and crying for no reason.

Other ways of preventing allergies are:

No smoking, drinking alcohol or taking medication and do not use gas appliances in a closed room. No painting or decorating in the house or painting the baby's equipment inside the house.

Use homeopathic or herbal toothpaste. Avoid fluoride.

Use non-biological washing powder and avoid fabric softener, toxic cleaners like bleaches, insecticides and herbicides

Use mineral water instead of tap water with all its added chemicals.

Avoid processed and junk foods and everything made from them. It has been found that some newborn deaths are due to damage done to the pituitary gland in the brain as a result of a diet high in sugar. This causes overactivity of certain enzymes which in turn damages the pituitary.

If you are really well-organised, you will detoxify your body, have a period of eating exceptionally well and drink tonic herbs such as red clover and nettles before becoming pregnant. Folic acid to prevent birth defects should also be started prior to conception and continued for the first trimester. If you have come off the pill to become pregnant, it is especially important to follow this routine, as the contraceptive pill washes out too many nutrients which are important in pregnancy. It is never too late to start eating properly so even if you have been eating unhealthy food in your early pregnancy, your baby will benefit from the moment you make the changes. Read all the dietary recommendations in this book, as they are all designed to build health.

Supplements of value

- **Calcium** - 1000 mg with **magnesium** - 500 mg - from the 4th month for the baby's bones. Take these separated from food and other minerals, preferably at bedtime.
- **Vitamin C** - 500 to 1000 mg daily with citrus bioflavonoids.
- **Zinc** - 15 mg daily separately from any iron.
- **Folic acid** - 400 to 800 mcg daily for the first trimester; 5 mg is too high a dose.
- **Vitamin B6** - 20 mg daily as pyridoxal-5-phosphate. B6 will prevent nausea if taken with vitamin C and zinc. It also prevents muscle cramps and determines the child's later learning ability. Do not exceed this dose as a routine - more is not better.

- **Vitamin A** - 2,000 IU with **Vitamin D -** 400 IU as fish oil. Beta carotene is better than vitamin A if you take higher doses.
- **Vitamin E** - 100 IU or up to 600 IU you have varicose veins
- **Kelp** - for iodine.
- **GLA as evening primrose oil -** 1,000 mg daily or half dose **borage oil.**

Most of these can be found in a pregnancy supplement along with other B vitamins and very important trace minerals like selenium, manganese and chromium.

Zinc - If the mother does not have enough zinc, the newborn may suffer inconsolable crying, poor weight gain, skin rashes or dermatitis, poor feeding and frequent loose stools. For her part the mother may feel unable to cope and be depressed. Zinc protects against malformations, dyslexia, undescended testes, a weak immune system and damage due to alcohol. However it must be taken separately from iron as the latter reduces the absorption of zinc from the intestines. It should also be taken at a different time from calcium. A 1985 study, found that pregnant women have 30% lower serum zinc than other women.

Folic acid - This should not be in too high a dose as it depletes zinc and vitamin B12. The correct dose is 400 to 800 mcg. If it is too high, there is a greater risk of birth complications. It can also lead to fever, hives, itching, a slow foetal heartbeat and respiratory distress. Over 1 mg daily is not recommended for epileptics as it may increase the likelihood of seizures.

Calcium - This must be taken separately from iron foods and supplements as it reduces iron absorption. Iron absorption from human milk is 48% and from the cow's variety, 19.5%. One interesting study showed that when calcium was added to human milk to reach the same levels as that contained in cow's milk, iron absorption from the human milk reduced to 28%. Calcium citrate and calcium phosphate were found to inhibit iron absorption by 49% and 62% respectively when taken with iron foods. When milk or cheese is taken with an iron food the absorption of the mineral is reduced by 10 to 60%.

Magnesium is always taken with calcium as the two work hand in glove for bone formation. However, low foetal magnesium is also associated with low birth weight which implies this mineral is necessary for normal foetal growth.

Iron - After reading the many studies on iron and pregnancy a certain pattern emerges. Serum iron, ferritin and haemoglobin levels are low in the early months of pregnancy, whether or not supplements are taken. One study found that the absorption of iron from food was only 7% at twelve weeks, 36% at twenty-four weeks and 66% at thirty-six weeks. Four months after delivery, absorption was down to 11%. Therefore pregnancy stimulates the absorption of iron in the mother's body exactly when needed and it makes no difference whether or not supplements are taken. It is much better to obtain iron from food than from pills. The following herbs are a good source of iron and may be taken in pregnancy: nettles, dandelion, alfalfa, yellow dock and fennel.

Vitamin E - High doses of this vitamin will often prevent a threatened miscarriage - wild yam root will do the same. Vitamin E will also prevent varicose veins at 600 IU daily, but do stop taking this as delivery approaches or the placenta may be too firmly stuck to the uterus. Premature birth is sometimes due to low levels of this vitamin in the infant. It does not pass the placenta easily and is destroyed by iron supplements in the mother's diet.

Essential fatty acids - These come in the form of nuts and seeds, soya beans and oily fish. A lack of these important nutrients means that the inflammatory prostaglandins are not kept in check. This is a prime cause of a lack of foetal growth and poorly developed immune and nervous systems. Eat oily fish three times a week unless you are vegetarian in which case you should eat two or more tablespoons of flaxseeds daily.

Sudden infant death syndrome (SIDS)

Although this is not part of pregnancy, it is at this stage that the syndrome can be prevented.

Infants who die of SIDS are deficient in vitamin C, B6 and iodine according to the independent discoveries of two doctors - Dr. Archie Kaloikerinos in the mid-60's in Australia and Dr. K. Fred Klenner in the United States from the 1950's onwards. Sometimes low selenium is also an issue. Those who die of SIDS in the form of heart attacks are deficient in vitamin B6 resulting in clogged blood vessels with fatty deposits. All these nutrients need to be given to the mother during pregnancy and then the child must be breastfed so that it continues to receive the vital nutrients. Dr. Kaloikerinos recommends 5 to 15 g of vitamin C daily but this seems unnecessarily high.

Iodine can be taken as seaweed in the diet of the mother or kelp tablets on a daily basis. If the infant is low in this mineral, its thyroid hormone will be deficient. Vitamin B6 has to be taken in the active form - pyridoxal-5-phosphate (P-5-P), as the infant cannot convert regular B6 (pyridoxine). The latter can cause B6 deficiency and subsequent damage to the nervous system. The signs of vitamin B6 deficiency in the mother are fluid retention, leg cramps and mood swings, depression or skin complaints. Anything over 25 mg daily which is suddenly withdrawn at delivery could lead to infant convulsions. It may also shut down the flow of breast milk if continued too close to delivery. If the infant is breastfed at birth withdrawal will not occur as vitamin B will still be available through the milk and can be slowly reduced in the mother's diet.

If a child is to be bottle fed after birth, both doctors recommend that vitamin C be given at the rate of 100 mg daily per month of age until it is getting 1000 mg daily at ten months old. If there is some diarrhoea at any stage, it means that the tissues are saturated: cut back to the level where it stops. Active vitamin B6 (P-5-P) should also be added to the formula in trace amounts, together with zinc at 0.5 mg per month of age up to 5 mg at ten months and iodine as kelp flakes in the formula. Both these pioneer doctors completely eradicated SIDS from their medical practices with this protocol. Fish oil should also be given to an infant who is drinking formula rather than breast milk.

You may think it impossible for an adult to be so deficient in vitamin C, B6 and iodine but a huge study in the United States has concluded that people eating a moderately healthy diet are below the RDA levels in many nutrients. RDA levels do nothing to build health; they just prevent serious disease.

Many other studies have investigated the reasons for SIDS and all have some validity. For instance, low levels of vitamin E and selenium have been related to this condition and it is a fact that mother's milk contains six times more selenium and twice the vitamin E that is found in formulas. It has also been postulated that if a mother's iodine is low in pregnancy, the infant is unable to make adequate amounts of thyroid hormone. Again, selenium has been implicated, as this mineral is important for the metabolism of thyroxine. Both very low and very high soil levels of selenium appear to trigger thyroxine deficiency in infants and a vitamin C deficit contributes to poor absorption of this mineral. One thing that is very clear from all of the above is that, not only are nutrients interlinked but their functions are dependent on a correct balance between one another.

Research in developing countries indicates that a low maternal iodine is associated with an infant mortality rate more than double the average. When iodised salt is added to the mother's diet, in those same areas, the mortality rate goes down by 50%. In developed societies, infant mortality is highest in regions where the soil is low in both iodine and selenium. This is the case in the south island of New Zealand. Researchers, examining the thyroid glands of 176 SIDS victims, reported that over 80% had evidence of low thyroid activity in life - the thyroid hormone is involved in many chemical reactions but is especially important for the maturing of lung activity and development of the nervous system in infants. At a conference on SIDS in Sweden in 1992, it was pointed out that SIDS infants have a malfunctioning nervous system which in turn has a detrimental effect on respiratory activity. If an infant is nutritionally deficient, SIDS can be triggered by exposure to infection or cigarette smoke, sleeping in a prone position or the shock of introducing toxic elements in the form of vaccines. Japanese research discovered that if DPT shots were delayed until children were two years old, the incidence of SIDS dropped by 50%. Where nutrient levels are critically low, the toxicity of the vaccine destroys the borderline stores and SIDS becomes a high risk problem. Sweden banned the whooping cough vaccine years ago and, along with Japan, is reputed to have the world's lowest infant death rate.

Cow's milk allergy has been propounded as a cause of SIDS and this is also a serious possibility. It has caused SIDS in animal studies.

Pre-eclampsia

In this condition, the blood pressure goes up, fluid collects in the legs and protein leaks into the urine. This type of hypertension and oedema is caused by sticky platelets in the blood. It is prevented by evening primrose oil, vitamins E and A, as well as adequate levels of calcium. These people have been found to have low vitamins E and A at 28 weeks. In an eclamptic fit, if intravenous vitamin E 10 to 12 g is given over twelve hours the child will be fine. Pre-eclampsia has been alleviated very quickly with magnesium 1 g and vitamin B6 1.5 g injected weekly for three weeks and then taken orally thereafter.

Low levels of various nutrients can lead to this condition. For instance where magnesium or calcium are too low, lead deposits increase and this can trigger pre-eclampsia. Low vitamin B6 is also a cause. This condition is recognised as one of poor nutrition. If you do start to develop signs of this potentially dangerous situation, take all the nutrients mentioned and increase your potassium levels with foods like potatoes, avocado, mango, peaches, banana, nectarine, all types of green vegetables, nuts, seeds and pulses.

Do not cut out salt in pregnancy - a little as flavouring is fine. If you do remove salt from the diet, it can trigger pre-eclampsia by stimulating an adrenal process that retains salt and therefore water. In other words, no salt causes a malfunction of the adrenal glands.

Herbs

There are a great many herbs which should not be taken in pregnancy but any mentioned in this chapter are safe and beneficial. Well known herbs like ginseng, hops, dong quai, golden seal, licorice, juniper, sage, southernwood, wormwood, basil, caraway, watercress, celery seed, nutmeg, sage, thyme, rosemary, marjoram and tarragon are all contraindicated in therapeutic doses. Of course the culinary ones may be used for flavouring.

Pregnancy tonics

Red raspberry leaf and **nettles**. Raspberry leaf tones the uterus by relaxing the muscle so that it can function better. It does not cause or strengthen contractions. Many herbalists prefer squaw vine to raspberry leaf, but the two may be combined so that delivery will be full term, safe and easy. Nettles provide vitamin K for the birth, together with many other nutrients. It cleanses the kidneys, and has an astringent effect on haemorrhoids.

Pregnancy sickness

Fennel, peppermint, spearmint, chamomile, meadowsweet or **raspberry** leaf teas are all helpful. **Wild yam** root is especially good - make it into a tea or take tablets.

Threatened miscarriage

Wild yam root prevents a threatened miscarriage. Make it into an infusion and drink 50 ml (2 oz) every 30 minutes. You can also mix equal parts **false unicorn** and **cramp bark** or **black haw** and make this into an infusion and drink a cup every four hours. Do all this until the initial danger has passed. False unicorn tones the uterus and cervix and is perfectly safe to take throughout pregnancy - especially where the cervix is too relaxed. Wild yam, cramp bark or black haw stop the uterine spasm so one of these herbs will be very important in the early stages.

Once the initial risk of miscarriage is over, it is wise to continue with some preventative treatment. I suggest wild yam tablets 1 to 2 g twice daily or 5 ml of the tincture. The safe dose is much higher than this. Tablets are preferable, as the tincture sometimes causes nausea. False unicorn is most important and the suggested dose is 1 to 2 g (tablets) or 2 to 5 ml (tincture) three times daily. Take black haw throughout your pregnancy if spasms continue to be a feature - one cup daily of an infusion or buy tablets and take 1 to 2 g two to three times daily. Tincture is also very effective and the suggested dose is 5 ml at the same frequency as the tablets.

Women who tend to miscarry may be deficient in the mineral selenium, which can lead to DNA damage. Selenium is an antioxidant and should be taken with beta carotene, vitamins E and C. Homocysteine levels are also normally elevated in those who miscarry recurrently, so folic acid, vitamins B12 and B6 should be routinely included.

In a 1996 study carried out by the University of Rome the blood levels of coenzyme Q10 were evaluated in 483 pregnant women. When this antioxidant was low, an increased risk of miscarriage was found. Normally coenzyme Q10 levels rise with each succeeding trimester, but in those who experienced contractile activity, the levels were significantly lower than in women who did not have any problems.

Varicose veins

Oatstraw or **nettle** infusion - one cup twice daily.

Hypertension

Passion flower, hawthorn berries, lime flowers and **skullcap**. Mix in equal parts and make an infusion; one cup twice daily.

Essential oils

Some oils are not safe to use in pregnancy and some are used only when delivery is approaching. Please do not experiment without knowing what you are doing. The oils mentioned here are safe and in fact, of benefit in pregnancy.

If feeling anxious or stressed, a massage with **neroli** or **frankincense** is wonderful and in insomnia, try some **lavender** with these herbs. Varicose veins are helped with **cypress** and **lemon;** oedema will improve with **rose** and **orange** or **lemon** mixed together. **Jasmine** relieves the pain of childbirth, but is not used beforehand. **Sage** and **nutmeg** oils may be used only in the last two weeks of the pregnancy: two drops of each in a carrier oil massaged into the tummy to tone the uterine muscle and prepare it for delivery.

Homeopathy

6C two hourly when necessary:

Arsenicum - for vomiting throughout pregnancy. Averse to the thought and smell of food. Complete loss of appetite and worry the baby will die as it is not eating. Anxious, restless and exhausted.

Asarum - for constant nausea and vomiting which is worse after food; even vomits water.

Sepia - for nausea with an unpleasant bitter taste which is worse from 3.00 to 5.00 p.m. Milky coloured mucus or bile vomited. Empty 'ball' feeling in the pit of the stomach. Hungry, yet the thought or smell of food makes the mother feel sick. She feels better after eating but must force herself to eat. Constipated, exhausted, irritable and may have backache.

Sulphur - for nausea throughout pregnancy, but little vomiting. Faintness at 11.00 a.m. and more nausea. Craves beer.

Ipecac. - for constant nausea and vomiting, especially if vomiting bile.

Kali carb. - for waves of nausea, but seldom vomiting. Cannot tolerate the feeling. Worse if anxious.

Colchicum - for violent nausea and vomiting when attempting to eat - feels faint with the need to eat, but the smell of food is disgusting - especially eggs and meat. Dry retching is frequent.

Nux vomica - for nausea and retching in the morning. Miserable and cranky until the afternoon. **Anacardium** has the same characteristics but is better for eating. Nux is a good remedy for indigestion in later pregnancy.

Pulsatilla - for nausea in the evening which improves in the night; a first choice remedy for varicose veins and haemorrhoids.

Nat. phos. - for nausea with a sour taste. Hunger after vomiting.
Symphoricarpus - for severe nausea and vomiting, aversion to all food, better lying on the back. The smell of food is repulsive. May need to take 200C potency.
Nat. mur. - averse to bread, fat and slippery food. Dislikes or craves salt.
Petroleum - for heartburn. Constant eating keeps nausea at bay. Averse to meat and fat. Worse with cabbage.

For threatened miscarriage

Dose with 30C hourly until your doctor arrives.
Arnica - if caused by a fall.
Belladonna - bearing down pains in the vagina, especially in the first trimester. The condition comes on suddenly. Passing clots followed by bright red bleeding. Hot, dry skin but no thirst. Backache, throbbing headache. Oversensitive to touch, light, noise and movement.
Sabina - especially in the first trimester. Pains start in lower back and move around to the pubic area. Pains are shooting and knife-like. Passes clots, haemorrhages bright red blood and has bearing down pains which are reduced if flat on the back.
Secale - especially for the first trimester. Haemorrhage without pain but the blood is dark in colour. Better if standing up and worse with heat. Timid and fears death.
Viburnum op - for cramping pains that radiate down the thigh. Left side worse than right. Dark spotting or mild bleeding only. Irritable and wants to be left alone.
Sepia - especially for the second trimester. Bearing down pains that feel as though everything is falling out. 'Ball' sensation in anus. Tired, weak, exhausted, averse to loved ones and sex. May have the dark face pigmentation. Very easily stressed and prone to difficult births.
Pulsatilla - intermittent bleeding which gets worse. The blood is dark and the pains like cramps.

Secale - at about the third month, cramping burning pain.

Sabina - uterine pain which extends down the thighs. Bright red blood which is partly clotted. Worse for the least movement.

Ipecac. - if very weak, bright red blood loss, vomiting and cramping pains.

Others

Go to antenatal classes so that you learn how to cope with breathing correctly and with pain. If you are well-prepared, you will be able to stay tuned in to your baby throughout the labour. It will need your constant reassurance and love.

Remember to take gentle exercise such as walking and swimming several times a week and to rest whenever you feel tired. The hormonal changes will cause a degree of fatigue. Relaxation techniques, visualisation and pregnancy yoga classes are all of great value and you should practise one of these three times a week. It will not only refresh you but will play a part in producing a contented, calm baby.

Conclusion

Having read all of this book, it will now be clear that the body is indeed self-healing if harmful elements are removed and the correct nutrients provided. There are natural means for restoring any type of hormonal imbalance. Sometimes specific vitamins or minerals are required to replace deficiencies and sometimes a situation calls for a single herbal remedy to assist nature in making far-reaching hormonal changes. Other women find that they have to deal with their hormone imbalance by a change in lifestyle or a different way of reacting to stressful situations.

The physical, emotional and spiritual bodies are interdependent: the well-being of one determines the health of the others. It is truly a matter of recognising where the problem originates and then taking the appropriate action to bring hormonal harmony and happiness into your life.

Bibliography

Infertility

Abraham, G.E., Hargrove, J.T., *Medical World News*, March, 1979.

Alternatives in Health, vol. 1, issue 1, June/July, 1995.

Carlsen, N.E. et al., "Evidence for decreasing quality of semen during the past 50 years", *BMJ*, 305, 1992.

Dawson, E.B. et al., "Sperm swim strongly after vitamin C therapy", *JAMA,* A249, (20) May 27, 1983.

Kumamoto, Y. et al., "Clinical efficacy of mecobalamin in treatment of oligospermia. Results of double blind clinical study.", *Acta Urol Japan*, 34, 1988.

Manomi, A. et al., "Coenzyme Q10 concentrations in normal and pathological human seminal fluid", *Journal of Andrology*, 15(6), 1994.

Schachter, A. et al., "Treatment of oligo-spermia with the amino acid arginine", *J Urol*, 110(3), 1973.

Sharpe, R.M., Skakkeback, N.E., "Are oestrogens involved in falling sperm counts and disorders of the male reproductive tract?", *Lancet,* 341, 1993.

Tikkiwal, M. et al., "Effects of zinc administration on seminal zinc and fertility of oligospermic males", *Indian J Physical Pharmacol,* 31(1), 1987.

Vitali, G. et al., "Carnitine supplementation in human idiopathic asthenospermia: clinical results", *Drugs exptl Clin Res,* 21, 1995.

Werbach, Melvyn R.,M.D., *Nutritional Influences on Illness*, Third Line Press, 1988.

PMS, endometriosis, menorrhagia and dysmenorrhoea

A Textbook of Natural Medicine, John Bastyr College Publication, 1985.

Abraham, G.E., "Primary dysmenorrhoea", *Clin. Obstet Gyn.,* 21, 1978.

Abraham, G.E., "Nutritional factors in the etiology of the premenstrual tension syndromes", *J Repro Med.,* 28, 1983.

Abraham, G.E., Hargrove, J.T., "Effects of Vitamin B on premenstrual syndrome. A double blind cross over study.", *Infertility,* 3, 1980.

Abraham, G.E., Lubran, M.M., "Serum and red cell magnesium levels in patients with pre-menstrual tension", *Am J Clin Nutr,* 34, 1981.

Barr, W., "Pyridoxine supplements in the pre-menstrual syndrome", *Practitioner,* 228, 1984.

Biskind, M.S., "Nutritional deficiency in the etiology of menorrhagia, cystic mastitis, PMS and treatment with vitamin B complex", *J Clin Endocrinology and Metabolism,* 3, 1943.

Brayshaw, N.D., Brayshaw, D.D., "Thyroid hypofunction in premenstrual syndrome", *NEJM,* 315, 1986.

Butler, E.B., McKnight, E., "Vitamin E in the treatment of primary dysmenorrhoea", *Lancet,* 1, 1955.

Cohen, J.D., Rubin, H.W., "Functional menorrhagia; treatment with bioflavonoids and vitamin C", *Curr Ther Res*, 2, 1960.

Cunnane, S.C., Horrobin, D.F., "Placenta linoleic and gamma linolenic ameliorate - the gross effects of zinc deficiency", *Proc Soc Exp Biol Med,* 164, 1980.

Deutch, B., "Menstrual pain in Danish women correlated with low omega 3 poly-unsaturated fatty acid intake", *European Journal of Clinical Nutrition*, 49, 1995.

Dittmar, F.W., Bohnert, K.J. et al., "Premenstrual syndrome treatment with a phyto-pharmaceutical", *TW Gynakol*, 50, 1992.

Downing, I., Hutchon, D.J.R., Poyser, N.L., "Uptake of arachidonic acid by human endometrium. Differences between normal and menorrhagic tissue", *Prostaglandins*, 26, 1983.

Facchinetti, F. et al., "Oral magnesium successfully relieves premenstrual mood changes", *Obst and Gyn*, 78, 1991.

Fine, B.P. et al., "Influence of magnesium on the intestinal absorption of lead", *Envir Res*, 12, 1976.

Goci, G.S., Abraham, G.E., "Effect of nutritional supplements on symptoms of pre-menstrual tension", *J Rep Med.*, 83, 1982.

Goci, G.S. et al., "Dietary patterns of patients with pre-menstrual tension", *J Appl Nutr*, 34, 1982.

Goldin, B.R. et al., "Oestrogen excretion patterns and plasma levels in vegetarian and omnivorous women", *New Eng J Med*, 307, 1982.

Horrobin, D.F., "The role of essential fatty acids and prostaglandins in the pre-menstrual syndrome", *J Repro Med.*, 28, 1983.

Horrobin, D.F. et al., "Abnormalities in plasma essential fatty acid levels in women with pre-menstrual syndrome and with non-malignant breast disease", *J Nutr Med*, 2, 1991.

Hudgins, A.P., "Vitamins P, C and niacin for dysmenorrhoea therapy", *West J Surg and Gyn.*, 62, 1954.

Lewis, G.J., "Do women with menorrhagia need iron?", *BR Med J*, 284, 1982.

London, R.S. et al., "The effect of alpha-tocopheryl on pre-menstrual symptomatology; a double blind study", *J Am Coll Nutr*, 2 1983.

London, R.S. et al., "Evaluation and treatment of breast symptoms in patients with the premenstrual syndrome", *J Repro Med*, 28, 1983.

Penland, J.G., Johnson, P.E., "Dietary calcium and manganese effects on menstrual cycle symptoms", *Am J Obstet Gyn*, 168, 1993.

Piesse, J.W., "Nutritional factors in the pre-menstrual syndrome", *Int Clin Nutr Rev*, 4, 1984.

Powell, A.M. et al., "Menstrual PGF2 alpha, PGE2, and TXA2 in normal and dysmenorrheic women and their temporal relationships to dysmenorrhoea", *Prostaglandins*, 29(2), 1985.

Rees, M.C.P., Anderson, A. et al., "Prostaglandins in menstrual fluid in menorrhagia and dysmenorrhoea", *Br J Obst & Gyn*, 91, 1984.

Shafer, N., "Iron in the treatment of dysmenorrhoea; a preliminary report",

Sherwood, R.A., Rocks, B.F., Stewart, A., Saxton, R.S., "Magnesium and the pre-menstrual syndrome", *Ann Clin Bio-chem.*, 23, 1986.

Taymor, M.L., Sturgis, S.H., Yahia, C., "The etiological role of chronic iron deficiency in production of menorrhagia", *JAMA*, 187, 1964.

Werbach, Melvyn R.,M.D., "Nutritional Influences on Illness", *Int J Alt & Comp Med*, July, 1992.

Fibrocystic breast disease

A Textbook of Natural Medicine, John Bastyr College Publications.

Abrams, A.A., "Use of vitamin E in chronic cystic mastitis", *New Eng J Med.*, 272, 1965.
Band, P.R. et al., "Treatment of benign breast disease with vitamin A", *Prev Med*, 13, 1984.
Ernst, V.L. et al., "Effects of a caffeine free diet on benign breast disease; a randomized trial", *Surgery*, 91, 1982.
Eskin, B.A. et al., "Mammary gland dysplasia in iodine deficiency", *JAMA*, 200, 1967.
London, R.S. et al., "Endocrine parameters and alpha tocopheryl therapy of patients with mammary dysplasia", *Cancer Res*, 41, 1981.
Minton, J.P., "Caffeine and benign breast disease", *JAMA*, 254, 1985.
Peters, F. et al., "Serum prolactin levels in patients with fibro-cystic breast disease", *Obstet Gyn*, 64, 1984.
Polson, D., "Polycystic ovaries - a common finding in normal women", *Lancet*, 1, 1988.
Pye, J.K. et al., "Clinical experience with drug treatments for mastalgia", *Lancet*, 2, 1985.
Werbach, Melvyn R.,M.D., *Nutritional Influences on Illness*.

Acne

A Textbook of Natural Therapies, John Bastyr College Publications.
Anderson, J.A.D., Stokoe, I.H., "Vitamin A in acne vulgaris", *BMJ*, 2, 1963.
Leung, L., "Pantothenic acid deficiency as the pathogenesis of acne vulgaris", *Medical Hypothesis*, 44, 1995.
McCarthy, M., "High chromium yeast for acne?", *Medical Hypothesis*, 14, 1984.
Michaelson, G., Juhlin, L., Ljunghall, K., "A double blind study of the effect of zinc and oxytetra-cycline in acne vulgaris", *Br J Dermatol*, 97, 1997.
Michaelsson, G. et al., "Erythrocyte glutathione peroxidase activity in acne vulgaris and the effect of selenium and vitamin E treatment", *Acta Derm Venerol*, 64, 1984.
Michaelsson, G. et al., "Effects of oral zinc and vitamin A in acne", *Arch Dermatol*, 113, 1997.
Michaelsson, G. et al., "Serum zinc and retinol binding protein in acne", *Br J Dermatol*, 96 (3), 1977.
Snider, B., Dieteman, D., "Pyridoxine therapy for pre-menstrual acne flare", *Arch Dermatol*, 110, 1974.

HRT and menopause

Bain, C.W., Willet, C.H., et al., "Use of post-menopausal hormones and the risk of myocardial infarction", *Circ*, 64, 1981.
Barrett-Connor, E., "Post-menopausal oestrogen and the risk of breast cancer", *Int Clin Rev*, Jan, 1995.
Bennett, F.C., Ingram, D.M., "Diet and female sex hormone concentrations: an intervention study for the type of fat consumed", *Am J Clin Nutr*, 52, 1990.
Berkgvist, L, et al., "The risk of breast cancer after oestrogen and oestrogen-progestin replacement", *NEJM*, 5, 1989.
Bewley, S., Bewley, T.H., "Drug dependence with oestrogen replacement therapy", *Lancet*, 339, 1992.
Bonnar, J. et al., "Coagulation system cahanges in post-menopausal women receiving oestrogen preparations", *Post Grad Med J.*, 52, 1976.
Briggs, M.H., "Mega dose vitamin C and metabolic effects of the pill", *BMJ*, 283, 1981.
"Cancer - is the war being lost?", *International Journal of Alternative and Complementary Medicine*, Aug, 1995.

Gow, S., MacGillvary, I., "Metabolic, hormonal and vascular changes after synthetic oestrogen therapy in ophorectomised women", *BMJ*, 2, 1971.
Grant, Dr. Ellen, *Sexual Chemistry,* Cedar, 1994.
Grant, Dr. Ellen, "Hormonal mayhem", *What Doctors Don't Tell You*, vol. 5, no. 5, 1994.
Grant, Dr. Ellen, "Long-term dangers of hormonal treatment", *Lancet*, April 9, 1994.
Hoover, R. et al., "Menopausal estrogens and breast cancer", *NEJM,* 295(8), 1976.
Hunt, K., Vessey, M., McPherson, K., "Mortality in a cohort of long term users of hormone replacement therapy: an updated analysis", *Br J Ostet Gyn.,* 97, 1990.
Inman, W.H.W. et al., "Thrombo-embolic and the steroidal content of oral contraceptives", *BMJ,* 203, 1970.
Psaty, Bruce M., et al., "A review of the association of estrogens and progestins with cardio-vascular disease in post-menopausal women", *Arch Int Med*, 153.
Shapiro, S., "Oral contraceptives - a time to take stock", *NEJM*, 315, 1986.
Skrabenek, P., "False premises and false promises of breast cancer screening", *Lancet*, Aug 10, 1985.
Stadel, B.V., "Oral contraceptives and cardio-vascular disease", *NEJM*, 305, 1981.
Steinberg, K.K., Smith, S.J., Thacker, S.B., Stroup, D.F., "Breast cancer risk and duration of oestrogen use: the role of study design in meta analysis", *Int Clin Rev.*, Jan, 1995.
Thorgood, M., et al., "Is oral contraceptive use still associated with an increased risk of fatal myocardial infarction?", *Br J Ostet Gynae*, 98, 1991.
Vessey, M.P., "Female hormones and vascular disease - an epidemiological overview", *Br J Fam Plan*, 6, 1980.
Wilson, P.F.W. et al., "Post menopausal oestrogen use, cigarette smoking and cardio-vascular morbidity in women over 50", *New Eng J Med.*, 313, 1985.
Whitehead, M., Stevenson, J., et al., "Dependence and oestrogen replacement", *Lancet*, 339, 1992.
Wright, Jonathan V.,M.D., "The oestrogen quotient", *Int Clin Nutr Rev.*, July, 1991.
Ziel, H.K., Finfel, W.D., "Increased risk of endometrial carcinoma among users of conjugated oestrogens", *NEMJ*, 293(23), 1975.

Menopause

Adlerdcreutz, H. et al., "Dietary phyto-oestrogens and the menopause in Japan", *Lancet*, 339, 1992.
Gazan, H.A., "The use of vitamin E in treatment of the menopause", *NY State Med J.,* May 15, 1952.
Hain, A.M., Sym, J.C.B., "The control of menopausal flushes by vitamin E", *BMJ*, ii 8-9, 1943.
Ishihara, M., "Effect of gamma oryzanol on serum peroxide levels and climateric disturbances", *Asia-Oceania J Obstet Gyn*, 10, 1984.
McLaren, H.C., "Vitamin E in the menopause", *BMJ*, 2, 1949.
Nutri Centre, Park Crescent, London - Reports on research in various countries.
Smith, C.J., "Non hormonal control of vaso-motor flushing in menopausal patients", *Chic Med*, Mar 7, 1964.
Werbach, Melvyn R.,M.D., *Nutritional Influences in Illness*.

Wilcox, G. et al., "Oestrogenic effects of plant foods in postmenopausal women", *BMJ,* 301, 1990.
Phyto-therapy. A Text Book of Natural Medicine, John Bastyr College Publications.
British Herbal Pharmocopoeia 1983.
Burton, Robert, *The Language of Smell,* 1976.
Christopher, Dr. John R., *School of Natural Healing,* Christopher Publications 1976.
Grieve, Mrs. M., *A Modern Herbal,* Penguin.
Mills, Simon Y., *The Essential Book of Herbal Medicine,* Arkana 1991, Planta Med Publications.
Tisserand, Robert, *The Art of Aromatherapy,* The C.W. Daniel Co. Ltd.
Weiss, Rudolf Fritz, M.D., *Herbal Medicine,* Beaconsfield Publishers, 1988.

Flower essences

Bach, Edward, *The Bach Flower Remedies.*
Scheffer, Mechthild, *Bach Flower Therapy,* Thorsons, 1986.
White, Ian, *Australian Bush Flower Essences,* Bantam Books, 1991.
Williams, R., *A Physicians Handbook on Orthomolecular Medicine,* Keats, 1977.

Nutrition and weight loss

A Textbook of Natural Medicine, John Bastyr College Publications.
Astrup, A., "Dietary fibre added to a very low calorie diet reduces hunger and alleviates constipation", *Int J Obes,* 14, 1990.
Bieler, H., *Diet Is Your Best Medicine,* Bantam Books, 1978.
Bland, Jeffrey, *Medical Application of Clinical Nutrition,* Keats, 1984.
Brown H., *Protein nutrition,* Charles C. Thomas Publishers, 1974.
Bulbrook, P.D. et al., "Breast cancer in Britain and Japan: plasma oestradiol-17B oestrone and progesterone and their urinary metabolites in normal British and Japanese women", *Eur J Cancer, vol. 12, 1976.*
Cheraskin, E., Ringsdorf, W.M., Clark, J.W., *Diet and Disease,* Rodale Press, 1968.
D'Adamo, Peter, N.D., "Gut ecosystem dynamics 111", *Townsend Letters for Doctors,* Aug/Sept, 1990.
Dickinson, L.E., et al., "Estrogen profiles of oriental and caucasian women in Hawaii", *NEJM,* 291, 1974.
Dulloo, A.G. and Miller, D.S. "The thermo-genic properties of ephedrine/methyl-xanthine mixtures; animal studies", *Am J Clin Nutr,* 43, 1986.
International Clinical Nutrition Review, 1990-1995.
Leung, L., "Pantothenic acid as weight reduction agent, fasting without hunger, weakness and ketosis", *Medical Hypothesis,* 44, 1995.
Messina, M.V., Messina, K., *The Simple Soya Bean and Your Health,* Avery Publishing Group, 1994.
Nutrition Almanac, McGraw Hill, 1979.
Oettie, G.J. et al., "Glucose and insulin responses to manufactured and whole food snacks", *AJCN,* 45, 1987.
Pfeiffer, C., Banks, J., *Total Nutrition,* Simon & Schuster, 1980.
Pfeiffer, Carl C., *Mental and Elemental Nutrients,* Keats Publishing, 1975.
Roger J. Williams, *Biochemical Individuality,* Bantam Books, 1978.
Rudolph Ballentyne, *Diet & Nutrition. A Holistic Approach.* Himilayan International Institute, 1978.
Thompson, J.K. et al., "Exercise and obesity; etiology, physiology, and intervention", *Psycol. Bull.,* 91, 1982.

Trowell, H. et al., *Dietary Fiber, Fiber Depleted Foods and Disease*, AC Press, New York, 1985.
Vasselli, J.R. et al., *Obesity; Present Knowledge in Nutrition,* 5th edition, Nutrition Foundation, Washington D.C., 1984.
Wolever, T.M.S., *The Glycemic Index*, World Review of Nutrition and Diet, 1990.
Yudkin, John, *Pure White and Deadly, the Problem of Sugar,* Davis Poynter, 1972.

Pregnancy

Arnaud, J., Prual, A., Preziosi, P., et al, "Effect of iron supplementation during pregnancy on trace element (Cu, Se, Zn) concentrations in serum and breast milk from Nigerian women", *Ann Nutr Metab*, 37, 1993.
Ashwell, M., "Fatty acids status and infant development", *BNF Nutr Bull.*, 19, 1994.
Barrington, J.W. et al., "Selenium deficiency and miscarriage: a possible link", *Brit J Obst and Gyn*, 103, 1996.
Cherry, F.F. et al., "Low plasma zinc levels were found in women with toxaemia", *Am J Clin Nutr*, 34, 1981.
Dawson, E.B., Kelly, R., "Calcium, magnesium and lead relationships in pre-eclampsia", *Am J Clin Nutr*, 51, 1990.
Foster, H.D., "Cot death and iodine and selenium imbalance", *Int Clin Nutr Rev,* July, 1992.
Foster, H.D., "Sudden infant death syndrome and iodine deficiency: geographical evidence", *J Orthomolecular Med*, 3 (1968).
Franz, K.B., "Magnesium intake during pregnancy", *Magnesium*, 6, 1987.
Guillarte, T.R., "Vitamin B6 and cognitive development: recent research findings from human and animal studies", *Nutr Rev*, 51 (7) 1993.
Hambridge, K.M. et al., "Zinc nutritional status during pregnancy; a longitudinal study", *Am J Clin Nutr,* 37, 1983.
Hattersley, Joseph G., "Stopping crib death", *Int J Alt & Comp Med*, September, 1994.
Kimura, M., Sakai, K., "Acellular pertussis vaccines and fatal infections", *Lancet*, April 16, 1988.
Money, D.F.L., "Vitamin E and selenium deficiencies and the possible aetio-logical role in the sudden infant death in infants syndrome", *NZ Med J*, 71 (1970).
Nettleton, J.A., "Are n-3 fatty acids essential nutrients for fetal and infant development?", *J Am Diet Assoc*, 93, 1993.
Noia, Guiseppe, et al., "Coenzyme Q10 in pregnancy", *Fetal diagnosis and therapy*, 11, 1996.
Sadeh, M., "Action of magnesium sulphate in the treatment of pre-eclampsia eclampsia", *Stroke*, 20, 1989.
Scholl, T.O. et al., "Low intake during pregnancy, its association with pre-term and very pre-term delivery", *Am J Epidemiol*, 137, 1993.
Schuster, K. et al., "Vitamin B6 status of low income adolescent and adult pregnant women and the condition of their infants at birth", *Am J Clin Nutr*, 34, 1982.
Sutton, R.V., "Vitamin E in habitual abortion", *BMJ*, October 4, 1958.
Truswell, A.S., "Nutrition for pregnancy", *BMJ*, July, 1985.
Villar, J. et al., "Epidemiological observations on the relationship between calcium intake and eclampsia", *Int J Gyn Obstet*, 21, 1983.
Werbach, Melvyn R.,M.D., *Nutritional Influences in Illness*.

Vaginitis

A Textbook of Natural Medicine, John Bastyr Publications.
Dolomore, B.A., et al., "Selenium status of Christchurch infants and the effect of diet", *NZ Med J*, 105, 1992.
Holmes, K.K., "The chlamydia epidemic", *JAMA*, 245, 1981.
Keller, van Siyke K., "Treatment of vuvo-vaginitis candidiasis with boric acid powder", *Am J Ob Gyn*, 141, 1981.
Liebman, Bonnie, "Baby formula: missing key fats?", *Nutr Action Health Letter*, Oct, 1990.
Maneksha, S., "Comparison of povidone iodine (betadine) vaginal pessaries and lactic acid pessaries in the treatment of vaginitis", *J Int Med Res*, 2, 1974.
Miles, M.R. et al., "Recurrent vaginal candidiasis - importance of an intestinal resevoir", *JAMA*, 238, 1977.
Riss, M., Weiler, G., Benker, G., "Comparative histological and hormonal studies of the thyroid gland with special reference to sudden infant death (SIDS)", *J Leg Med*, 96, 1986.
Vontver, L. et al., "The role of gardnerella vaginalis in non specific vaginitis", *Clin Ob Hyn*, 24, 1981.
Willinger, M., "State of the art conference on SIDS, Gothenburg, 1992", *Acta Paediatrica Suppl*, 389.
Willmott, F. et al., "Zinc and recalcitrant trichomoniasis", *Lancet*, 1, 1983.

Homeopathy

Benjamin, H., *Everybody's Guide to Nature Cure*, Thorsons, 1981.
Boericke, W., *Materia Medica with Repertory*, Boericke and Tafel, Phil 1927.
British Homeopathic Journals.
Clark, J.H., *Clinical Repertory*, Homeopathic Publishing Co., London 1904.
Clark, J.H., *Dictionary of Materia Medica*, (3 volumes), Homeopathic Publishing Co., London, 1925.
Coulter, Catherine R., *Portraits of Homoeopathic Medicines*, North Atlantic Books. 1986.
Foubister, Dr. Donald, *Tutorials on Homeopathy,* Beaconsfield Publishers 1989.
Kent, James Tyler, *Lectures on Homeopathic Philosophy*, 1979.
Kent, J.T., *Materia Medica*, 2nd edition, Sinha Roy, Calcutta, 1970.
Lessell, C.B., *Homeopathy for Physicians*, Thorsons, 1983.
Lockie, Dr. Andrew, *The Family Guide to Homeopathy*, Penguin, 1989.
Tyler, Margaret L., *Homeopathic Drug Pictures*, Health Science Press, 1952.
Wright, Elizabeth, 1977, *Brief Study Course in Homeopathy*.

Stress

Alberti, K.G., Nattrass, M., *Lancet*, 2:25-9, 1977.
Blackmores Prescribers Reference for Botanicals 1986.
Chopra, Deepak, *Perfect Health*, Harney Books, 1990.
Dubos R., *Man Adapting*, Yale University Press, 1966.
Fink, D.H., *Release from Nervous Tension*, Unwin, 1945.
Kermani, Kai, *Autogenic Training*, Souvenir Press.
Pfeiffer, Carl C., *Mental and Elemental Nutrients,* Keats Publishing, 1975.
Rainey, J.M. et al., *Psychopharmac Bull*, 20(1):45-9, 1984.
Scheffer, Mechthild, *Bach Flower Therapy*, Thorsons, 1986.

Selys, H., *The Stress of Life*, McGraw Hill, 1956.
Shaw, D.L. et al., "Management of fatigue: a physiologic approach", *Am J Med Sci*, 243:758, 1962.
Siegal, Bernie, *Peace, Love and Healing*, Rider, 1990.
Siegel, Bernie, *Love, Medicine and Miracles.*
Weiss, R.F., *Herbal Medicine*, Beaconsfield Publishers, 1988.
Wheeler, F.J., *The Bach Remedies Repertory*, C.W. Daniel, 1952.
White, Ian, *Australian Bush Flower Essences*, Bantam Books.
Wood, Clive Dr., *Say yes to life*, Dent, 1990.

Osteoporosis

Abraham, G.E., "The importance of magnesium in the management of primary post-menopausal osteoporosis", *J Nutr Med*, 2, 1991.
Alternatives for the Health Conscious Individual, vol. 4, no. 6, Dec, 1991, with the following references:
J Repro Med, 83:28: 446-64. Proc Natl Acad Sci 83; 80; 7646-9. N Eng J. Men 82; 307; 1542-47. J. Clin Endocrin Metab 82; 55; 102-107. Hawaii Med J 77; 36; 39-77. Int Clin Nutr 84; 54-81. J. Repro Med 83; 28; 449-464. J Am Coll Nutr 84; 3; 351. N Eng J Med 90; 322; 802-9. Lancet 90; 3 36 (8726); 1327.
Cannata, J. et al., "Effect of acute aluminium overload on calcium and parathyroid hormone metabolism", *Lancet*, 1, 1983.
Cauley, J. A. et al., "Endogenous oestrogen levels and calcium intakes in post menopausal women", *JAMA*, 260, 1988.
Christiansen, C. et al., "Prediction of rapid bone loss in post menopausal women", *Lancet*, 1, 1987.
Christiansen, C., et al., "Uncoupling of bone formation and resorption by combined oestrogen and progestogen in post menopausal osteoporosis", *Lancet*, Oct, 1985.
Coats, C., "Negative effects of a high protein diet", *Family Practice Recertification*, 12, 1990.
Diesendorf, M., "The health hazards of fluoridation: a re-examination", *Int Clin Nutr Rev.*, no. 2, 1990.
Eaton-Evans, Jill, "Copper Supplementatition And The Maintenance Of Bone Mineral Density In Middle-Aged Women", *et al, The Journal Of Trace Elements In Experimental Medicine, 1996; 9:87-84.*
Editorial - "Citrate for calcium nephrolithiasis", *Lancet*, 1, 1986.
Editorial - "Fluoride and the treatment of osteoporosis", *Lancet*, 1, 1984.
Ellis, F. et al., "Incidence of osteoporosis rate in vegetarians and omnivores", *Am J Clin Nutr*, 25, 1972.
Gaby, Alan R., "Progesterone; oral versus transdermal", *Townsend Letters for Doctors*, Aug/Sept, 1994.
Gaby, Alan R., Wright, J.V., "Nutrients and bone health", *JAMA*, 4, 1988.
Hartard, Manfred, "Effects On Bone Mineral Density Of Low-Dosed Oral Contraceptives Compared To And Combined With Physical Activity", *et al, Contraception, 1997; 55:87-90.*
Kynast-Gales, S.A., Massey, L.K., "Effect of caffeine on circadian excretion of urinary calcium and magnesium", *Int Clin Nutr Rev*, Oct, 1995.
Law, M.R. et al., "Preventing osteoporosis", *BMJ*, 383, 1991.
Lee, C.J. et al., "Effects of supplementation of the diets with calcium and calcium rich foods on bone density of elderly females with osteoporosis", *Am J Clin Nutr*, 34, 1981.

Licata, A. et al., "Acute effect of dietary protein on calcium metabolism in patients with osteoporosis", *J Geron*, 36, 1981.

Marsh, A.G., "Cortical bone density of adult lacto-ovo-vegetarian and omnivorous women", *J Am Diet Assoc.*, Feb, 1980.

Marsh, S. et al., "Vegetarian lifestyle and bone mineral density", *AJM*, 82, 1987.

Massey, L .K., "Dietary salt, urinary calcium and kidney stone risk", *Nutritional Reviews*, 53,5. 1995.

Nielsen, F.H., "Boron, overlooked element of potential nutrition importance", *Nutrition Today*, Jan/Feb 1988.

Nielsen, F.H., Hunt, C.D., Mullen, L.M., Hunt, J.R., "Effect of dietary boron on mineral oestrogen and testosterone metabolism in post-menopausal women", *North Dakota Academy of Science*, April, 1987.

Prior, J.C., "Progesterone and its relevance for osteoporosis", *Bull for Physicians*, Mar, 1993.

Riggs, B.L. et al., "Effect of fluoride treatment on the fracture in post menopausal women with osteoporosis", *New Eng J Med*, 322, 1990.

Riss, B.R. et al., "Does calcium supplementation prevent postmeno-pausal bone loss?", *NEJM*, 316, 1987.

Travers, R.L., Rennie, G.C., Newnham, R.E., "Boron and arthritis, the result of a double blind pilot study", *J Nutr Medicine*, 1, 1990.

Van Papendorp, D.H., Coetzer, H., Kruger, M.C., "Biochemic profile of osteoporotic patients in essential fatty acid supplementation", *Int Clin Nutr Rev*, Oct, 1995.

INDEX